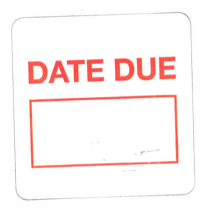

DATE DUE

Asperger Syndrome

Asperger Syndrome

Natural Steps toward a Better Life

Suzanne C. Lawton, N.D.

Foreword by Judyth Reichenberg-Ullman, N.D.

Complementary and Alternative Medicine
Chris D. Meletis, Series Editor

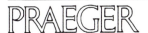

Westport, Connecticut
London

Library of Congress Cataloging-in-Publication Data

Lawton, Suzanne C., 1955–
   Asperger syndrome : natural steps toward a better life / Suzanne C. Lawton ; foreword
by Judyth Reichenberg-Ullman.
         p. ; cm.—(Complementary and alternative medicine, ISSN 1549–084X)
      Includes bibliographical references and index.
      ISBN-13: 978–0–275–99178–4 (alk. paper)
         1. Asperger's syndrome.   2. Asperger's syndrome—Alternative treatment. [DNLM:
1. Asperger Syndrome.   2. Adolescent.   3. Adult.   4. Child.   5. Complementary
Therapies. WS 350.6 L425a 2007]   I. Title.   II. Complementary and alternative
medicine
   RC553.A88L395   2007
   616.85′8832—dc22   2007023402

British Library Cataloguing in Publication Data is available.

Library of Congress Catalog Card Number: 2007023402
ISBN-13: 978–0–275–99178–4
ISSN: 1549-084X

First published in 2007

Praeger Publishers, 88 Post Road West, Westport, CT 06881
An imprint of Greenwood Publishing Group, Inc.
www.praeger.com

Printed in the United States of America

The paper used in this book complies with the
Permanent Paper Standard issued by the National
Information Standards Organization (Z39.48–1984).

10 9 8 7 6 5 4 3 2 1

This book is intended to provide the reader with information only. As noted throughout
the text, individuals should consult appropriate health care practitioners knowledgeable
in the field of natural medicine prior to pursuing any particular course of treatment.

Names and identifying facts have been changed for all case studies included within this
book so that individuals who may be described in the case studies will not be recognizable.
Any similarities between the case study descriptions and actual, living persons are purely
coincidental.

The publisher has done its best to make sure the instructions and/or recipes in this book
are correct. However, users should apply judgment and experience when preparing recipes,
especially parents and teachers working with young people. The publisher accepts no
responsibility for the outcome of any recipe included in this volume.

Contents

Series Foreword

Dr. Suzanne Lawton and the growing number of physicians that embrace health care from a truly integrative approach are pioneering the way for the next quantum leap in significant advances in both academic and clinical medicine. With the support of the National Institutes of Health (NIH) and National Center for Complementary and Alternative Medicine (NCCAM) and funding from both private and public sectors the appreciation for the integration of health care education and delivery is becoming a greater reality.

There is no more important time for all health care providers to embrace the concept of "individualized patient oriented wellness." Thanks to the work of Dr. David Eisenberg and similar studies we now know that Americans are allocated billions of discretionary dollars to seek out what used to be termed "alternative medicine" approaches. Yet what was once considered fully "alternative" is becoming integrated, as evidence grows, into the mainstream. The first step in true integration is to realize that health care is a continuum that is both fluid and dynamic.

The nearly ten-fold increase in autism over the last twenty years demands that this epidemic serves as a unifying force for all fields of medicine to work seamlessly in resolving what many consider the ultimate "coal miner's canary" of modern society. It is only through the concerted efforts of the whole health care and research community that the formulation of hypotheses relative to the increased prevalence, potential etiologies, diagnostics, and treatment options can most expeditiously be addressed. With our public and private school systems, families, and social services fully entrenched in this epidemic and the current trending of statistics, the only option is prevention and early intervention.

This work on Asperger's syndrome is an important contribution that provides a platform for health care provider and patient alike to proceed with a heightened level of awareness, insights, and literally a head start in establishing a working foundation to meet the unique needs of each patient as they participate in the lifelong journey of health care, which should be with the advent of an integrated approach that would more accurately be termed "wellness care."

Chris D. Meletis
Series Editor

Foreword

Asperger Syndrome (AS) has, as Dr. Suzanne Lawton so correctly reminds the reader, baffled Dr. Hans Asperger and baffles parents, children, physicians, and other health care practitioners, researchers, and others to this day. We cannot seem to agree on the cause or even, universally, on the diagnosis, much less the treatment. Auditoriums full of angry, impassioned, sometimes desperate, parents have gathered to berate the apparent lack of concern on the part of governmental institutions regarding mercury-laden vaccine preservatives. Families spend inordinate amounts of time, energy, and financial resources on any number of health care approaches for their Asperger children. So many affected children, so many questions, and so few answers.

We can agree that the number of children, and adults, diagnosed with AS has risen to the point that many would consider to be epidemic. The current estimate is one out of every 150 children in this country. Though, coinciding with the removal (relatively speaking) of thimerosal in most childhood immunizations, the numbers appear to be diminishing; the incidence is said to be growing considerably in China, where we are now exporting those earlier batches of preserved vaccines.

Given the groundbreaking discovery of a gene associated with autism, we may agree on some genetic component. Yet to come to light is exactly how that hereditary tendency might make this group of children and adults more susceptible to environmental influences.

We can agree that AS embraces a complex, curious, and often confusing constellation of symptoms. And that, despite their sometimes superior intelligence and efforts to adapt to our neurotypical society, these children and adults experience tremendous challenges—physical, emotional, social, academic, and sensorial. Despite their efforts to do the best they can, they frequently find themselves misunderstood and ostracized.

So, now that there is more widespread consensus that AS does in fact exist, is more prevalent than Hans Asperger would have ever imagined, and that it is indeed a serious problem for parents, adults, families, educators, and for our society, what do we do about it?

You may have heard the expression, "If you are a hammer, everything looks like a nail." Professionals addressing the dilemma of AS tend naturally to use the therapies or approaches with which they are most familiar. Conventional physicians choose pharmaceuticals; complementary and alternative physicians generally opt for DAN (Defeat Autism Now)! Protocol: nutritionally oriented practitioners recommend the gluten-free/casein-free (GF/CF) diet. And, so it goes, with each team, so to speak, rallying around a particular treatment protocol or set of protocols. This book, on the other hand, offers a cornucopia of well-researched and effective natural alternatives presented in an open-minded, practical manner.

I suppose that I am prejudiced toward this book already because I am a licensed naturopathic physician (N.D.) of twenty-four years. So much of what I appreciate about naturopathic medicine is embodied in this book by Dr. Lawton. Naturopathic students learn, from day one, about the principle of vis medicatrix naturae, the healing power of nature. As an N.D., I genuinely believe that, despite insults, imbalances, and insults that the organism, if nudged gently in the direction of healing, has the ability to heal itself. This is far different from the concept of the "anti's"—antibiotics, antifungals, antihistamines, and immunosuppressants, etc. Naturopathic doctors, as you will be reminded again and again as you read this book, trust that natural healing is not only possible, but the most sane and commonsense way to heal ourselves. Through a healthy lifestyle that includes breathing fresh air, ingesting whole, live foods, natural therapies and lifestyle, and a healthy, loving family and environment, we can lead our AS children to healing—safely, gently, and naturally.

Dr. Lawton speaks from her own clinical experience. It is clear that she respects and understands her AS patients in a way only someone who has worked with numerous adults and patients with this diagnosis can. She recounts their stories and shares with the reader their successes with compassion and care. Her approach is fresh, wide in scope, and quite practical. As a naturopathic physician specializing in homeopathy, I find Dr. Lawton's breadth in considering such a wide variety of natural, sensible approaches to treating AS patients to be impressive and useful. There is enough of a variety of recommendations in this book to suit any parent seeking a natural approach for their AS child, or any adult with AS.

I appreciate that Dr. Lawton does not mince words concerning the importance of an organic, sugar, and pesticide-free diet for anyone with AS. The fewer noxious chemicals that we put into our own and our youngsters' bodies, the less we need to worry about removing them in the future. Whether you are curious about how to alter your family's diet to promote health and well-being, how to heal your child's gut naturally, what to make of the current wave of chelation therapies, or how homeopathic remedies can produce dramatic healing, you will find it all in this book.

And lest you think that last is least, I cannot help but put in a final plug for homeopathy. An excellent adjunct to the other approaches described in this book or, for those children who cannot tolerate the taste or side effects of other therapies, a stand-alone modality. Safe and gentle enough even for pregnant moms, newborns, the elderly, and, yes, children and adults with AS and sensory hypersensitivity, homeopathy can be ideal for this population.

I congratulate Dr. Lawton on her excellent, user-friendly work, and hope that this book finds its way into the hands of parents, adults, and professionals concerned with AS. I know that I will be recommending this book to my patients!

Judyth Reichenberg-Ullman, N.D., L.C.S.W.
Coauthor of A Drug-Free Approach to Asperger Syndrome and Autism:
Homeopathic Care for Exceptional Kids, at http://www.drugfreeasperger.com.

Preface

When I started writing this book, I set out to offer a more natural, science-based medical treatment option to the Asperger community. Along the way, things changed. Hearing story after story of Asperger children and adults struggling to fit into what the general population has defined as normal, I began to see that this issue, like all issues, has two sides. Gradually, I recognized Asperger Syndrome as a different way of thinking based on variations in the brain, similar in many aspects to speaking a foreign language. To successfully navigate through his life, the challenge for the person with Asperger Syndrome is twofold. First, he should learn the "language" that the majority of people speak where he lives, while *not* forgetting his own. This means learning the basic acceptable forms of behavior within his community, whether that community is the classroom, the workplace, or a restaurant. In short, as Liane Holliday Willey so succinctly entitled her book, it means "Pretending to be Normal" in some circumstances. And second, along with all the non-Asperger folks, he/she should work to establish balance in his/her own life. For the person with Asperger Syndrome this includes learning to not overreact, to be less anxious, and to be content with who and what he/she is. Though this is easier said than done, it is what this book is all about.

There is no one single solution which helps every solitary person with Asperger Syndrome. Each person's situation is unique and will require a specific combination of treatment options. However, within these pages there is enough information to devise a plan that will help your situation or guide you as you work with a medical professional.

This book is dedicated to all the Asperger square pegs trying to fit into round holes, and to my patient husband and my incredibly supportive children. It's also dedicated to all the AS and non-AS people who have encouraged me in this process.

CHAPTER 1

Asperger Syndrome: What It Is and What It Isn't

Dr. Hans Asperger sank back into his chair, shook his head, and sighed. He had been poring over his reports on thirty-four children with peculiar mannerisms each night for weeks, and still could not understand why they behaved this way. They couldn't seem to interact normally with others and many were overly sensitive to sound, taste, smell, or touch. They were highly anxious and often had trouble staying focused on what was said to them. Some, with their flat affect and monotone voice, appeared slow-witted and dull. Why did these children have these strange symptoms? Was it neurological, or psychological, or both? How many of them were out there? What could be done to help them? And what would happen when these children grew up to become adults? Dr. Asperger closed his eyes and sighed again. He needed answers.

Asperger Syndrome (AS) has baffled scientists ever since Dr. Asperger first started studying these children in 1944. Over the next sixty years, people with AS have been labeled schizophrenic, devoid of emotion, mentally challenged, incapable of leading successful, healthy, productive lives, emotionally disturbed, insane, phobic, and incurable. But whatever label the experts tried to apply, it never seemed to fit. How could a person who appeared so dull-witted write so eloquently or finish a computer project in half the time as his fellow workers? How could a person devoid of emotion devote their professional life to helping children in special education school programs or create inspiring artwork?

Along with the labels the psychiatric community attached to this group, came the driving impetus to fix these people. A group of people who think and perceive the world completely differently from the average person needed to be educated to think and perceive the world like everyone else.

Not surprisingly, AS was soon classified as a mental illness and was often confused with schizophrenia. Since AS was initially examined in the very limited context of these children's behavioral abnormalities, some important questions were missed. Were there any physical symptoms that the children shared? And was there a familial component? Could this condition be passed via the genes or was this behavior unique and isolated?

Over sixty years later, we have some answers to these questions. With the advantage of studying thousands rather than thirty-four cases, we know considerably more about AS than the pioneering scientists. We know that Asperger Syndrome is a continuum ranging from very severe cases to very mild ones. In the severe cases, the person may continue to live with his parents, be institutionalized, or be in government-assisted living situations. Simple decisions like food or clothing purchases are beyond their capability. In some cases, they are able to hold down lower level part-time jobs. At the other end of the spectrum are the mild cases that go largely unnoticed in the general population. These people have jobs, families, and may live right next door.

If we look at AS in a larger context, we can see a more complete picture. Practitioners who treat children with AS often see parents with some similar traits. One of the parents may rarely socialize but prefer the company of his family. One of the parents might have few if any hobbies and instead be focused fairly intensely on his job. One of the parents may be using prescription medicine for anxiety. If asked, they will often report an eccentric relative, maybe an Aunt Ramona or an Uncle Henry, who has even stronger AS characteristics. Aunt Ramona either says nothing for long periods of time or blurts out embarrassing and often personal statements at family get-togethers. Uncle Henry talks at great length about a single topic, which is usually his work, and very often will have little to no interest in whatever you are saying. At a family event, Aunt Ramona might abruptly leave after thirty minutes or stay way too long. Uncle Henry isn't exactly rude, but you wonder why he acts so peculiar, doesn't bathe often, dresses strangely, and always seems so ill at ease. These adults share similar symptoms with the children Dr. Asperger studied in the 1940s. Could there be a link? Could Asperger Syndrome simply be a name for an intensified version of a variation in thought process that has always existed?

Asperger Syndrome is characterized by a combination of significant social, sensory, attention, and anxiety challenges. A simple weekend trip to the mall could feel like going to a rock concert—a lot of noise, people, and confusion. Afterwards, they might be worn out and need to recuperate. The person with AS may be clumsy, unable to do sports, or even master handwriting, have some obsessive-compulsive behaviors, and often overreacts to all sorts of situations, especially social events. They don't realize they are being rude or that their mannerisms are extremely distracting to others. They perceive their rudeness as being direct and their mannerisms, such as pacing or clapping, simply as ways to release energy. They have trouble relaxing and often fail to understand when others are joking. When significantly overstimulated by noise and people, they overreact and may have meltdowns at school or outbursts at work or at home. Many children and adults with AS may have an additional neurological condition called prosopagnosia or face blindness. While there are no firm statistics available to reflect just how many people with AS are affected, I have found that about 35–40 percent of my AS patients also have this condition. Just as it sounds, people with prosopagnosia can't remember faces. That means on the second day, Alex can't remember which of the fifteen other little boys in his class he played with on the first day. As an adult, Alex will have a hard time remembering one cousin's or in-law's face from another. He will, however, have learned to recognize characteristics and voices. This makes for very poor social interaction. But happily, while some AS traits seem so detrimental, others can be constructively channeled, resulting in a productive and happy child and adult.

For example, some people with either multiple AS traits or the diagnosis itself go on to join Mensa (an international organization for people with IQ's in the top 2 percent of the general population), win Nobel prizes, become successful writers, work in Silicon Valley, or become researchers in the space program at NASA. There are easily recognizable AS characteristics in scientists such as Nikola Tesla, a pioneer in the development of electricity, or Ludwig Wittgenstein, a famous Viennese/English logician and philosopher. Even Albert Einstein and Isaac Asimov had some AS traits. For people with AS, their single-mindedness and attention to detail allow them to stay focused on their specific area of research.

People with AS are often employed in technical fields and make excellent, if not particularly social, employees. They are the rare employees that see their job as an extension of themselves and therefore strive to do the best they can. When given some latitude, AS employees demonstrate remarkable problem-solving abilities. In their personal relationships, they are loyal, though not particularly demonstrative spouses who take on an extra project or chore for their spouse as a token of their affection than give a hug. Naively honest, most people with AS adhere to a strict sense of right and wrong.

Over sixty years ago, Hans Asperger described the syndrome as a mental illness and it has been treated as such ever since. One has to wonder if there are so many productive people with AS, why it continues to be treated as a mental illness—unless all the researchers are studying only the most severe cases. More recently, AS has been added to a group of related neurological conditions called the autism spectrum. The autism spectrum encompasses five main conditions: Autism, AS, Rett Syndrome, Pervasive Developmental Disorder Not Otherwise Specified (PDD-NOS), and Childhood Disintegrative Disorder. Some scientists and psychologists even add the increasingly common neurological condition, Attention Deficit (Hyperactivity) Disorder (AD(H)D) with this group, since the Autism Spectrum conditions invariably contain AD(H)D characteristics.

Research on the Autism Spectrum has focused on aspects such as the size of the head, the parts of the brain that are most affected, the onset of language skills, and what the most effective medications are to decrease the anxiety and increase the attention. The true nature of AS is so poorly understood that more than one medical journal compared the Asperger population with that of the severely mentally handicapped Down's Syndrome.[1] While there is little dispute that people with AS have characteristics that should be addressed by the mental health community, for many years the physical components of AS have been mostly ignored.

PHYSICAL CHARACTERISTICS OF ASPERGER SYNDROME

In 1998, Dr. Andrew Wakefield and his colleagues at the Royal Free Hospital in Hampstead, England, shook the psychiatric world with a surprising discovery. He identified an intestinal condition in autistic children, which he labeled autistic enterocolitis,[2] and he proposed that healing this intestinal condition would improve the psychological symptoms of these children. Most of the psychiatric community responded with derision and condemnation. But some, spurred by the challenge, made similar observations.[3,4] This confirmation opened the doors to other physicians looking for a set of common physical denominators in the autistic population. The hope was that if there were physical symptoms that could be resolved, then that would help diminish the behavioral symptoms. And for a few thousand children with autism, this hope has become a reality. There is a similar challenge with AS. Practitioners like myself are seeing very definite physical patterns alongside these sets of behaviors. We see varying intestinal problems including stomachaches, chronic constipation or diarrhea, and fungal infections, which often stem from a history of frequent antibiotic use. Headaches are also common in AS children. In AS adults, the intestinal problems include more serious conditions such as irritable bowel syndrome (IBS), intestinal blockage, and various forms of colitis. Also in adults, the prolonged state of anxiety can result in high blood pressure and other heart conditions. In both groups, sleep disturbances, nervous mannerisms, and food allergies are routinely present.

In the mid-1980s, Dr. Doris Rapp, another trailblazer in the research of physical complaints causing behavioral changes, charged onto the scene. A pediatric allergist turned environmental medicine pioneer, Dr. Rapp recognized the connection between what children eat and how they behave.[5] Previously, the medical community saw food allergies only in relation to physical symptoms. Dr. Rapp disrupted medical mainstream assumptions when she introduced the idea that food could cause major behavioral changes—often for the worse. To demonstrate this, she brought some well-behaved children onto a popular television talk show. The children were given ordinary foods such as orange juice or peanut butter to which they were individually sensitive. In a matter of minutes, they became violent and disruptive. But Rapp didn't limit her research to food. Her work also demonstrates how significantly toxins routinely found in homes, offices, and schools, can affect mood and behavior.[6] Using her research model within the Asperger community, it's easy to see how food, household, and workplace affects both children's and adults' behavior. And happily, there have been similar positive results when removing the food and decreasing chemicals and toxic metals to which a person is sensitive. That means children who blurt out seemingly rude statements or the adult who overreacts to a simple request at work can maintain control if they avoid foods and chemicals to which they are sensitive. Imagine what this means in the school, work, or family life setting. But though extremely important, diet is just one tool in natural medicine to treat AS. In the last few years working with hundreds of patients, we are finding that natural medicine, which uses herbs, vitamins, homeopathy, and various nutrients, is making a significant difference in both the children and adult AS population.

CONVENTIONAL MEDICAL MODEL

Natural medicine centers on an individually focused medical model that works differently than conventional medicine. With conventional medicine, if someone is overreactive and acting inappropriately, she might be prescribed an antipsychotic or mood stabilizer, such as risperidone. Risperidone can be very effective in modifying these symptoms. It must be regularly monitored by lab work as it can harm the liver, an already compromised organ in people with AS. In some patients, there may be side effects such as dizziness, anxiety, headaches, dry mouth, menstrual abnormalities, abdominal pain, various skin conditions, and lethargy. In others, it partially, but not completely resolves the targeted symptom. While conventional medications can be very effective and don't require lifestyle changes like natural medicine, they rarely address underlying causes.

NATURAL MEDICAL MODEL

For the same condition, a natural physician would look at the person's diet, internal and external environment, and determine if there is an underlying condition such as hypoglycemia or lack of protein, which may be affecting his mood. He would then prescribe natural medicine supplements, a homeopathic remedy, herbs, a change in sleep and/or dietary changes—all of which are nontoxic and designed to resolve the unwanted behavior and improve the person's overall health. There is often a noticeable improvement in behavior within a week to two weeks, and some patients report feeling better even sooner. The goal with natural medicine is to heal the underlying condition and decrease the tendency toward the excessive behavior, not just to suppress it. Natural medicine will not cause dizziness, anxiety, mood changes, headaches, dry mouth, menstrual abnormalities, skin conditions, or lethargy.

Though some people think it is new to the medical community, natural medicine has been safely used by practitioners for hundreds of years and is becoming increasingly the focus of research centers around the world. It can be used in place of or alongside conventional medication. Despite the benefits of both conventional and natural medicine in addressing AS the condition frequently requires more than medical treatment. Most people with AS lead productive lives and need no intervention. For those who are more affected, it often helps if they have a better understanding of how the rest of the population thinks and even more importantly, how to interact reasonably smoothly with them.

Since the person with AS processes information differently, the social skills that the average person absorbs naturally as a child are foreign behaviors to the child and subsequent adult with AS. For example, the ten-year-old child with AS won't understand why it's rude to pull away from Grandma's hug while saying, "Grandma, you smell funny." That might be understandable behavior in a three-year-old, but not in a ten-year-old. Or the husband who doesn't understand that agreeing with his mother-in-law that her Thanksgiving turkey was a little dried out and burnt, was not a good idea. This means the parent either alone, or with the help of various therapists skilled in treating the AS population, must teach acceptable behaviors to the child. And it means that an adult with AS who wants to advance in his corporation or repair his relationship with his in-laws might benefit from social counseling, an AS mentor, or even a community college class on more appropriate social behavior. The integral role of AS-knowledgeable therapists will be discussed in detail in Chapter 5.

Once we treat the physical conditions with conventional or natural medicine and work with therapists on the behavioral symptoms, the overall AS symptomatic picture diminishes.

INCREASE IN ASPERGER SYNDROME

Over the last few decades there has been an increase in the diagnosis of AS. In 1993, the *Journal of Child Psychology and Psychiatry* reported that 36 per 10,000 children were diagnosed with AS.[7] This is an epidemic increase from the 0.6 per 10,000 figures presented by researchers Wing and Gould in 1979.[8] Was this symptomatic of previous underreporting or were there more cases? Some asserted that since AS is relatively new, doctors didn't know what to look for and therefore didn't report it. Others refuted this and blamed a host of probable causes including changes in lifestyle, environment, and diet for the increase. Christopher Gilberg, a professor of Child and Adolescent Psychiatry at Gothenburg University, the recipient of several scientific awards and one of the pioneers identifying particular genes involved with autistic characteristics, proposes that a milder form of AS exists among children in approximately 0.7 percent in the general population.[9] These children and their parents are productive, have less pronounced symptoms, and have stayed under the AS diagnostic radar. MRI scans of the brains of both AS children and their parents revealed similar atypical brain function.[10] Also supporting the familial tendency toward this condition, another study showed similar auditory patterns in both Asperger children and their parents, especially with their fathers.[11] An article in the *Journal of Autism and Developmental Disorders* found that in a hundred boys with AS, 50 percent of them had a person with an Autism Spectrum condition on the father's side.[12] Even comparing the level of amino acids, such as glutamic acid, phenylalanine, asparagine, tyrosine, alanine, and lysine, in the Asperger child with his family and then to non-AS families, revealed that the whole family had similar patterns to the AS child and different ones from the non-AS families.[13] While this research supports the familial tendency, it doesn't explain why each subsequent generation seems to have more pronounced symptoms. Perhaps external causes are affecting this static percentage, which Gilberg describes, and have caused an increase in the symptomatic picture.

Misdiagnosis

Some in the conventional medical community explained the increase in AS cases as a result of misdiagnoses. A 2001 article in *Advances in Psychiatric Treatment* said that the increase in Asperger diagnosis is the failure to correctly diagnose schizophrenia, high functioning autism, and other conditions on the autism spectrum.[14] In a practical sense, this seems a bit specious. There is a big difference between schizophrenia, in which a person talks to someone who doesn't exist, and Asperger in which the person doesn't talk to people who do exist. However, a more probable misdiagnosis is pyroluria. Pyroluria is a genetic blood disorder that scientists discovered over thirty-five years ago. Depending on the source, it is present in about 3–10 percent of the general population. Pyroluria has many symptoms, such as anxiety and social withdrawal, which overlap those of AS. This condition is important to consider and will be discussed more comprehensively later in the book. To make matters more confusing, mental health conditions such as bipolar disorder and depression can also simultaneously affect people with AS.

Environmental Influence

In the maverick forefront of probable causes for the increase in reported AS cases are environmental influences. There is substantial evidence that environmental toxins adversely affect both the human body and mind. It's easy to see how it can similarly exacerbate AS symptoms. For example, the common AS characteristic of mild inability to interact with others can become exaggerated given the right stimulus. Uncle Henry, who has always preferred a solitary cat as his only company and rarely socialized, now barricades himself and ten cats in his house. The same basic characteristic is now intensified into a pathology because of environmental influences.

While researching the effect of the environment on people, Dr. Doris Rapp coined the condition Allergy Tension Fatigue Syndrome (ATFS) to explain a series of mental, emotional, and physical reactions that correlate to the increased pollutants in our homes, workplaces, and schools. ATFS is a very comprehensive approach.[15] Some scientists, looking for a simpler explanation focused purely on heavy metal toxicity such as mercury, lead, and aluminum. Children and adults with autism and Asperger can have higher levels of these metals as well as toxic chemicals than the average person.[16] ATFS and heavy metal toxicity cause symptoms that overlap those of AS.

A 2001 article in *Pediatrics* medical journal that drew national attention studied a community of 75,000 people who had an incidence of Autism Spectrum conditions including Asperger Syndrome considerably higher than the national average.[17] The authors of the article safely declined to draw any conclusions because they found similar isolated increases in other studies. Their conclusion didn't stop conjecture from all fronts as to why there were so many cases in this community. An examination of the U.S. Environmental Protection Agency's list of EPA-Regulated facilities in the same zip-code listed a concrete company, dry cleaners, and a wood mill as spewing toxic substances in this community. A 1999 Environmental Protection Agency study reported that people living near plants where cement is processed, such as a concrete company, may inhale harmful airborne dioxins, arsenic, cadmium, chromium, thallium, and lead at levels especially dangerous to children.[18] A common emission from wood mills, dioxins are actually a group of compounds that can cause changes in normal development and learning disorders. Perchloroethylene (Tetrachloroethylene) leaking from poorly controlled dry cleaners targets the nervous system and the liver. While without more evidence, specific conclusions can't be drawn, it does suggest that there can be a factor involved with this town's unusually high number of AS cases. But air pollution is just part of the environmental picture.

Dietary Influences

Another way some experts argue that environmental influences are affecting neurological conditions such as AS cases is with food. Over the last five decades our food supply has undergone massive changes. Our diets are heavy in highly processed foods lacking in nutritional value. Much of the food in restaurants and on our tables has additives and preservatives that may extend the shelf life, but may have a completely different effect on human life. I strongly urge my patients to eat organic food whenever possible. One particularly resistant patient became a strong supporter after he ate an organic steak on a trip to Montana. He couldn't believe how great it tasted compared to his steak from the supermarket. And despite the five-vegetables-a-day recommendation, if we peeked into the majority of homes during mealtime, we would see few adults and even fewer children eating their veggies. I still have to explain to a few patients each month that catsup and French fries don't count as vegetables. Fast food, frozen dinners, and pre-made food consumption continues to be high despite how much research shows the value of whole fresh foods and the marginal value of overprocessed ones. Several minerals, especially zinc, have been depleted from our soil for decades. A daily multivitamin and mineral supplement isn't enough to compensate for the loss of nutrition, especially when that supplement is laden with sugar, food coloring, shellac, or chemicals such as magnesium stearate to make it move smoothly through the machinery. What's more, the insecticides and pesticides, which are routinely sprayed on our crops and fed to our livestock, are not benign. Insecticides and pesticides target the nervous systems of bugs and rodents and may be affecting the human nervous system as well when found in the foods we eat.[19] If, as this argument suggests, these alterations to our food may be exaggerating the AS symptoms, it seems logical to simply avoid these substances rather than take medications and risk potential side effects and damage the liver.

While we understand AS more than earlier researchers, there is still so much more to learn. There are so many varying presentations that one solution doesn't fit all cases. In the following chapters, we'll explore both scientific research and clinical experience of a poorly understood condition. This book presents solid evidence-based understanding of the condition, along with practical natural treatments with supportive research and clinical experience that can be implemented at home or under the guidance of a natural medicine provider. There are so many options that it might seem a little overwhelming. Take your time, start with one or two things, see what works and then add or delete. These treatments are powerful, though gentle. Unlike most books on AS, this one addresses both adults and children with AS, since they share the same characteristics though the presentation may differ in intensity. AS is often a family affair and the same medical principles work for both age groups.

Most importantly, I hope we can end the negative stigma of AS as a mental illness and instead recognize it as an alternate pattern of thought processing, which has existed for hundreds of years, recently exacerbated by lifestyle and environmental influences. Since he was treating children with what seemed as an aberrant condition, Dr. Asperger didn't look to the parents or family. If he had, he might have seen similar patterns in these adults. After all, these children must have gotten these neurological patterns from somewhere. And if he looked even harder, he may have seen similar patterns throughout society.

CHAPTER 2

What Asperger Syndrome Looks Like in Children and Teenagers

Most parents feel relieved and anxious when their child has been diagnosed with Asperger Syndrome (AS). They are relieved to know their child's behavior has a name but are also worried about what their child's life will be like. It often eases this apprehension to give an overall picture of what the condition looks like. This helps to explain the mannerisms and unusual thought patterns as well as aid the parents in understanding their child's own personality traits are versus AS characteristics. Depending on when your child was diagnosed, it can be helpful to know what AS looks like in younger children versus teenagers. Without a good understanding of the condition, parents may find themselves inundated with confusing AS variations such as the "little professor" and the "idiot savant" personas. Neither are really accurate portrayals of children with AS. Like any other condition, AS has extreme and mild, younger and older versions. Some Asperger children only exhibit their AS characteristics when under pressure. For others, the flat voice and the aversion to eye contact make it much more obvious. This chapter will give parents snapshots of many AS children. Some may be recognizable, others not. No two AS children are identical and no two AS children are completely dissimilar. Equally as important, this chapter will help explain the child's behavior. If parents understand the thought process, they can better counsel and help the child navigate what is for him overwhelming and alien.

After the relief and anxiety, the next thought that often floods the parents' minds after the diagnosis is wondering how their child got AS. What did they do wrong? The parents didn't do anything wrong. AS has a familial component, which means that the parents or close relatives will have similar characteristics. Parents often acknowledge some similarities but fervently deny the intensity of their child's symptoms. In the overwhelming number of cases, this is true. The children's symptoms are more severe than their parents. What has happened to alter children's nervous systems generation after generation? While there are no definitive answers yet, there are many possible environmental explanations. Our food supply is increasingly sprayed with insecticides and pesticides that target the nervous system of the insects and pests and may secondarily affect the human nervous system. Vaccinations may also be a factor both in the number and the preservative content of vaccinations. The air we breathe is increasingly contaminated with chemicals that adversely affect the nervous system. All these environmental influences will be discussed in detail in Chapter 8. It seems that a familial weakness in the nervous system can make this particular group more susceptible to adverse effects from environmental toxins than the general population.

AS CHILDREN: AGES ONE TO ELEVEN

Children with AS share some basic characteristics, which may vary in intensity from mild to severe. You will consistently see anxiety, signs of being frequently overwhelmed, nervous mannerisms, abrupt behavior changes, difficulty with change, a strong desire for routine, naiveté and innocence, discomfort with one or more sensory issues, a contentment with playing alone, poor eye contact, some obsessive-compulsive behaviors, some AD(H)D (attention deficit disorder with or without hyperactivity), intense fascination with a limited number of subjects, and both a social detachment and a delayed social development.

Most often I see two basic patterns for younger children. Either they have extreme personal boundaries and are shy and withdrawn, or they seem to have no boundaries and venture into others' space without invitation. Both will have huge anxiety issues, poor eye contact; both will lose control fairly easily when overstimulated; and both will be extremely literal.

Several books on AS often identify the "little professor" persona as the normal Asperger child. Within this group of AS children, there is often a flat affect of the voice, a lack of cadence, or natural rhythm to their speech. Anger may be expressed by a staccato effect alone rather than by pitch or volume. Enthusiasm is expressed by action rather than an excited voice. Even with AS children who have "normal" voices, when they are nervous, they tend to formalize their language. They may stop using contractions and start sounding like robots. I tend to see elements of that persona but rarely do I see a full-fledged little professor. Occasionally, I will see parents who foster this "little professor" persona. For example, they make the assumption that a child who can easily memorize and parrot various facts is somehow more intelligent than the next-door-neighbor's child who is playing with trucks. They bolster this difference by telling the "little professor" child he is special or somehow better than his non-AS counterpart. Sadly, these children seem to do extremely poorly in school compared to the AS child whose parents praise the factoid memory, while consistently encouraging the child to work on social skills. It's important for the parents to remember that their child will grow up and that it's essential that he develop essential social skills.

The second type of AS child has poor physical boundaries. This child will come up too close to other children or strangers. In school, they will just walk up and take a crayon from another child while that child is using the crayon. They can be very confused as to why this is inappropriate in other settings as well. For example, Bob, a bright and happy AS child with poor boundaries, scared his cousins in the pool with dunking games and rough play at a family get-together. Even with his cousins, and then his aunts and uncles, asking him to stop and eventually simply getting out of the pool to avoid him, he just didn't seem to understand what he was doing wrong. He would giggle and smile and finally wondered aloud why the other children were running away. His lack of social boundaries and inability to pick up social clues hindered any positive social interaction with his peers. Even worse, if this behavior isn't checked it can develop into unintentional bullying or can become dangerously violent.

HOME VERSUS PUBLIC

An interesting phenomenon that explains the frequently late diagnosis of many AS children is that there is a noticeable difference between their behavior at home versus at school or at church. Many parents note that the AS behavior is almost nonexistent, even with non-AS siblings, in the home setting. In the often much less stressful home environment, the AS characteristics are mild. Sometimes this becomes a problem with one parent denying that the behavior and disconnect even exists. Most often I see this with fathers, simply because they don't see the child in an environment outside the home as much as the mother. My advice to the parent reading this book is to be patient. Let the other parent take the child to Sunday school, to boy scouts, or even to school a few mornings. Actions speak considerably louder than words.

Innocence

One of the first things you notice about most children with AS is an innocence usually reserved for the very young. The AS child will appear years younger in social maturity than his non-AS counterpart. In fact, there is often a two-to-three-year social delay with most AS children. This results in the AS child being comfortable with younger friends. So, often you will see a six-year-old child playing happily with her four-year-old next-door neighbor rather than the neighbor's six-year-old sibling.

I often start my office visits asking the child about his favorite toys or games. This unleashes a beautiful heartfelt monologue in which the child earnestly attempts to share his passion for whatever the subject matter is. The old folk song "Puff the Magic Dragon," tells the story of a little boy whose favorite toy is an imaginary dragon. As the child grows up, he shifts his attention away from the dragon. Most AS children would be happy to continue playing with the dragon indefinitely. Some AS preteens and teenagers will even say, "I wish I could have stayed a child forever."

Routine

Coupled with the innocence is often a confusion that seems to dominate their actions and thoughts. While they prefer to conduct their lives with utmost simplicity and directness, they can't understand the changeability of the rest of the world. They tend to see the world in black and white. Toys should be played a certain way, and dinner routines shouldn't change. His one or two friends should always want to play the same games. Food should always be separated on the plate. Life should be consistent. That is why when an AS child goes traveling with family and deviates from his routine, the mother might bring his eating utensils along. The utensils aren't a security blanket in the usual context as there is no sentiment attached to these objects, but it does provide structure and consistency in an unfamiliar situation. As one eight-year-old frequently stated, "If everyone would just follow the rules, everyone's life would be easier." Without consistency, the Asperger child is out-of-sync with most of the rest of the world, which then leads to this confusion. With consistency, they can awkwardly but successfully proceed.

Sensory Issues

Sensory issues appear less consistent in the AS population. Some children may cry with touch, seem sound-sensitive, or have trouble eating certain textured foods; while for others this is less of a concern.

Kyle was an odd baby. One stranger remarked that Kyle looked like a Raphael painting, with beautiful contemplative eyes. While this initially seemed flattering, Kyle's mom was concerned that her child wasn't bonding. He cried every time his mom tried to hug him, except when she was feeding him. Fortunately for Kyle, he wasn't her first child. His mom didn't take it personally and accepted he was just an unusual baby. Realizing he needed to slowly get used to physical contact, she started off by giving him one-second hugs. Over time, she gradually lengthened the hugs and within a few months, Kyle was comfortable with physical contact.

For Kyle, his mom's initial hugs caused a sensory overload. He was able to decrease this overload when his attention was directed toward nursing, but not otherwise. His mom's gradual desensitization helped him better adapt to a world with touch.

Sensory issues are a common problem with AS children. Sometimes they are extremely obvious like revulsion for certain food textures and tastes, or aversions to crowds or loud noises, and at other times it is less apparent.

Eleven-year-old Tom refused to go to the mall—even when he had out-grown his clothes. When forced, he would seem as if he was having a panic attack and beg his mom to let him wait in the car. Puzzled by this behavior, his mom would have many talks with him to try to understand it. Tom didn't understand it himself and would just repeat that he hated malls. Looking for a pattern, she saw that Tom did fine in the library, but not in any large box stores except hardware stores. She began to see that the colors, smells, and noises of the mall overwhelmed him. The hustle and bustle of the shoppers seemed to make things worse. But if he was otherwise focused such as at a library or at a hardware store, he could decrease the sensory effect. Tom's mom discussed this with him and explained that he would need to overcome this sensory issue to become a successful adult. Like Kyle's mom, Tom's mom worked on desensitizing him and started him off with five-minute visits. They picked a store, went right to the young men's section, found and purchased one or two articles of clothing, and left. Ten years later, Tom still dislikes malls and prefers to shop online. But he can shop anywhere when he chooses.

These sensory issues can get amplified quickly. Sean, a curious three-year-old with AS, seemed fine in the car, but couldn't control himself at the supermarket. He would run up and down the aisles as fast as he could. Eventually, his mom realized that the lights, noise, and overall energy of the supermarket were over-stimulating to his nervous system. His running was just his way of releasing some of the increased stimulation. She used two tactics that seemed to work. First, she engaged Sean in every purchasing decision by keeping an ongoing dialogue with him. She was redirecting his attention and even more importantly, reducing the focus of his stimulation. Second, she changed the time she went shopping to either first thing in the morning or last thing at night when the store was empty. Another mother who employed this same technique soon realized that if she named a product and helped focus the child on obtaining that product, he often didn't even notice the candy five feet away.

Sensory overstimulation is much more difficult to address in the child's class-room. There, if the child is overstimulated, she will act out. Once upset, the AS child has a fairly slow recovery rate. It's as if their nervous system is struggling to regain balance. One solution seems counterintuitive for a person with poor social skills. But, if the child is allowed to sit off in a corner a little away from the other children, they have essentially developed a "safe" space and seem to have more control over their behavior by retreating to this space. And while this isn't meant as a solution for all children, it seems to work for some.

Empathy

A characteristic of AS children that has caused some controversy is the re-ported lack of empathy. An AS child may watch her friend fall on the playground and may not go over to see how she is. After talking with many AS adults I have discovered that they do feel empathy, but it is limited and delayed. They seem to need time to process emotions. In my experience with AS children, I find this true as well. If asked, "How do you feel about . . . ?" they will look blank and have to think for a while. Or they might realize something is wrong but simply don't know how to correctly express compassion. One three-year-old, when seeing his mom cry, walked up to her and poked her eyes and said, "No." It was as if he recognized crying was a sign of unhappiness, but thought that the cause was the tears rather than the situation. If an AS child is on the playground and witnesses another child fall, it is not obvious to them that the child might be in pain and need some comfort. Once the AS child has seen others comfort the fallen child, she will then know what to do. However, when they do have the appropriate response, it can seem stilted and affected. The AS child may seem to lack empathy and watch impassively as a child gets hurt.

Some AS children don't seem to recognize the moods attached to facial expressions of others or simply don't intuitively know how to respond. They can't always tell when a parent is upset or if they have just hurt a friend's feelings. Once the parent or friend tells them that they are upset, the AS child will often respond appropriately or quizzically. They are still trying to figure out what they did that caused the other person to be upset. This isn't malice, but a true inability to "read" the situation. Most parents don't see these characteristics in their children until the child is about four or five years old. This lack of response is one of the first clues to AS.

Anxiety

Asperger children are typically extremely anxious. Parents will notice this much more in public than at home. One of the earliest signs that most, but not all AS children have is the perpetually worried look on their faces. I have even seen this in babies who later were diagnosed with AS. Anxiety and fear manifest in many ways. The child may be excessively fearful of having his hair washed and take hours to calm down afterwards. One little girl responded to an accidental choking on a piece of food by not eating for several days. She was terrified of repeating the experience. Many AS children are terrified and yet drawn toward scary movies. A common theme is the fear of being hurt by others or by events such as hurricanes or earthquakes. Many AS children have developed coping strategies to neutralize fear. Some are healthy others are not. One little girl would very gently stroke her own arm two to five times to ground herself. A teenage boy would play thirty minutes of video games to take his mind off the fear and anxiety. Less healthy coping strategies are those who hit themselves and berate themselves for what appears as silliness in girls and cowardice in boys.

Eye Contact

Children with AS may act peculiar around other children and there is often poor eye contact. While children won't be able to explain it, several

AS adults have explained it to me that they avoid others' gazes as a way to decrease overstimulation. Simply put, other people's eyes are distracting to them. They lose their train of thought. So, it is not uncommon for a child to make eye contact, avert her eyes, make the statement, and then remake eye contact.

Stimming

"Stimming" or nonsexual self-stimulatory actions are less common in Asperger children versus truly autistic children. A parent can generally tell if the child is stimming as they will be in a world of their own and not really relate to others. For example, one child would place playing cards over an air-conditioning vent just to watch them fly around. Each time the card shot up, the child would do almost a complete body trembling of excitement. This behavior continued for over twenty minutes. A non-AS child may find the same thing entertaining, but for five minutes or so and would not experience a full body trembling of excitement. The atypical responses to sensory stimulation are called sensory integration dysfunction. Sometimes the dysfunction is minimal and frankly, not affecting the quality of that child's life and parents can resolve this on their own. In more severe cases, the child might need the services of professional therapists, especially occupational therapists, in both schools and private practice that are trained in treating this condition.

Hiding

AS children like to hide. Both the outgoing and shy AS child will try to squeeze into small spaces and may stay hidden for long periods of time. This differs from the normal childhood game of playing tent. Instead, the AS child will choose a quiet place (such as the living room sofa) to stretch out behind. They will not announce where they are but simply disappear. Often he will press himself firmly between the sofa and the wall. This comforts the child and appears to help the nervous system decompress from overstimulation. Sometimes, it isn't hiding as much as just getting into small places where the child can feel safe. This behavior can continue well into the teenage years.

Obsessive Behavior

In some AS children, there are elements of obsessive compulsive behaviors. It may be mild or extreme. It can range from rechecking and rechecking the van doors to excessive hand-washing or concerns about cleanliness. Sometimes this behavior can look like one thing and be another. One ten-year-old girl started washing her hands for one to two minutes at a time. Curious, her mom asked why she was doing this. "My hands are cold," was her innocent reply. It's important to investigate reasons before jumping to conclusions.

A related theme with AS kids is an intense fascination with one or two topics. The child becomes preoccupied with a subject and it becomes a source of pride for parents. Unfortunately, the child finds it difficult to communicate with others outside the parameters of his topic. And while this can seem harmless, once it is recognized the subject matter should gently be expanded.

> Six-year-old John loved jeeps. In fact, he had a scrapbook on jeeps and would talk about them each day. Sometimes, he would even go to the jeep dealership to touch and climb into the jeeps as well as pick up more brochures. Unfortunately, this fascination limited John's ability to talk with other people. Even though others would try to steer him away from talking about jeeps, he doggedly persisted. At first, others listened good-humoredly, then less so. Finally, John's dad came up with a solution. He talked with John to find out what John liked so much about jeeps. John liked the strength and power. So, John's dad got a book on military tanks. John read it. Then John's dad got a book on World War II and John read that. Over the course of a few months, John's dad broadened his interests from jeeps to tanks to World War II. John latched onto World War II for several years before refocusing onto other subjects. Over the years, John realized that he loved machines and eventually became a mechanical engineer.

By encouraging a related topic, John's dad helped John out of a potentially detrimental behavior pattern. Asperger children are high maintenance, but with intuitive and creative parents they can flourish and can lead productive happy lives.

Bossiness

Some AS children can become remarkably bossy. I see this in about 25–30 percent of the cases. These are generally the brighter AS children who are trying to control the situation. For example, a Brownie girl scout, whose mom was the troop leader, may boss the other little girls around in the group. If you ask the AS child, it will quickly be apparent that this behavior isn't as much to control the other children as an inappropriate role modeling. The AS child won't necessarily make the distinction that the mother is the leader and she is one of the troop. She identifies with her mother and considers herself a leader as well. Typically, this leads to a social alienation, which baffles the child. It is at this stage that the child must learn to change this behavior. The parents often think that simply saying, "Don't be so bossy," will help. The child often doesn't know that they are being bossy. Nor does, "You wouldn't want someone to treat you like that," seem to help. Instead, a careful reconstruction of behavior with role-playing seems to help the child amend this behavior. Often, if you appeal to the AS child's heightened sense of order and rules, it works much more effectively. Even though it requires a lot of effort on the parent's part, it will help the child considerably more than removing them from the situation and hoping for a better outcome the next time. With AS children, it's good to remember that they very often lack the ability to intuit correct social behavior. If you work via the AS child's intellect on learning the "rules" of social interaction, you will be giving them tools that they will take with them as an adult into the business world in which group interactions are often the norm. You will also help them get past their one-on-one comfort zone.

Unfortunately, "the rules" that many AS children love for others to conform to are often "their own rules." After hearing her father routinely complain about the messiness of the house, one AS ten-year-old girl devised a system for keeping the house clean with a rotation of chores. Despite her working mom's encouragement, she couldn't understand her siblings' or father's refusal to participate as her plan would have resolved the messiness issue. She didn't realize that when her dad spoke of a cleaner house, he wasn't offering to be involved in that process. The ability to comprehend that others have their own beliefs, needs, and intentions is called "theory of mind." Many AS children and adults lack this ability in varying degrees. However, with careful guidance they can develop it to some degree.

Friends

Both AS children and adults prefer one-on-one social interactions. In fact, most AS children are content and even flourish with a single friend. Problems can arise when AS children find that their friends have other friends. This confusion may show up in multiple ways. One AS child, confused that her special friend had another friend, climbed to the top of the school jungle gym and jumped down on top of the other friend. When asked why she did this, she didn't know. Fortunately for the AS child, it looked like an accident. Later, her mom sat down and carefully explained how people often have more than one friend and gave her strategies to deal with this. The child was then able to be friendly toward the other child as well. This social disconnect may be part of the abnormalities in neural circuitry in AS. Once the child understands, they can repattern more appropriate responses via an alternative circuitry.

Males versus Females

Statistically, there are more documented cases of AS in males than females. There are several reasons for this discrepancy. Boys are socialized differently from girls. Girls are taught from an early age to empathize. Similarly, there is more pressure on girls to conform to certain behaviors and avoid others. Initially, boys are given wide latitude in behavior but then dramatically curtailed when entering school. For the non-AS child, this transition takes a month or two. For the AS boy, this transition is a shock to their system and may take considerably longer. Again there is confusion. Why is this place called school so dramatically different from home? The teacher often doesn't know or doesn't have the time to help the AS child deal with new sounds, smells, or activities. The parents are often not aware of the difficulty, as the child will have trouble expressing himself. In short, school is change and sensory overload—the two things that can throw an AS child into increased anxiety and overreactivity.

Attention Issues

In 50 percent or more of children with AS, there will be some amount of attention deficit disorder (AD(H)D) with or without hyperactivity. Often, it is what the child is first tested for before she is diagnosed with AS. The child will hyperfocus on some subjects and completely tune out others. You might ask him to set the table and find him twenty minutes later completely engrossed in something else. Or you might repeat, "Dinner is ready," ten times to a seemingly deaf child absorbed in a book or a game. Though there are exceptions, this is not defiant behavior. The child has simply become distracted and must be brought back to the task. There are dozens of books written on strategies for treating AD(H)D. From firsthand experience as someone with AD(H)D and having raised a child with AD(H)D, one works with the jumbled flow rather than against it. I will hyperfocus for a few hours and then need to jump from one part of one task, to one part of another task. For example, as a child, I did part of my math homework, jumped over to reading, and then back to finishing up the math. This has allowed me to be extremely productive. It also didn't seem to affect my ability to do tests. However, I had a wonderful mother who while joking about me having "ants in my pants" as a young child, which was the old-fashioned description of a very active, restless child, still was able to help me become organized within the context of ADHD. The AS child is a square peg. Sometimes it's best not to try to push them into a round hole.

Bullying

Bullying is a serious problem that seems to plague AS children. With their extreme naiveté, they might just as well wear targets on their chests. These children often don't seem to realize they are being bullied. It is as if they are mentally and physically paralyzed in a situation in which they have no idea what is going on or what they should do. You will see this pattern in adults as well. When they are overwhelmed by a situation, their reasoning ability seems to shut down. These children are often uncoachable with snappy one-liners. And often teachers are so overtaxed by multiple students that the bullying may be noticed, but is often ignored. It may not be apparent to the adult that the AS child who is just standing there looking blankly around, is taking an emotional beating as badly as the one crying in the corner. Sadly, the bullied AS child may become the bully. It is critical to address this behavior. If the AS child has discovered bullying as a coping mechanism, it needs to be stopped before it becomes violent. A therapist can help address this. There are a couple of wonderful books on bullying, which I have included in the Appendices.

Paul, an extremely bright six-year-old male was wonderful around adults. His precocity and engaging manner masked the scary behavior he exhibited to other children and to himself. He was expelled from several day care centers for biting and hitting other children without remorse. Once old enough for school, he was quickly identified as a "special needs" child because of his aggressive behavior. Surprisingly, his high-powered executive father who was frequently away on business trips, didn't see or believe any accounts of this behavior and preferred to believe he was a slightly rambunctious little boy whom neither his mother nor the various teachers could handle. Sometimes, it can be hard for the parent who sees less of the child to recognize the seriousness of the situation.

EXTENDING THE ASPERGER SYNDROME CHILD'S COMFORT ZONE

Easing the child into the outside world is the arduous task of the parents. Many parents have done a great job in gently helping their child be less rigid. It's extremely important that this transition is done kindly and carefully. Like any condition on the autism spectrum, AS behavior can become even more extreme and autistic-like if the child feels unsafe. In fact, some AS children, because of their extreme sensitivity can develop a PTSD-like state, which can persist for years. One AS adult remembers that as an accomplished swimmer, she, at the age of five through eight years, was shunted along with her siblings to various competitions. For her siblings, these trips were exciting adventures. For her, despite multiple awards in the sport, the trips were terrifying experiences of too many people, too many smells, and too much noise. So much so that for the next twenty years, she had trouble smelling chlorine as it brought waves of memories of her sitting in the corner crying and trying to escape the noisy confusion of a swim meet.

Kent, another AS adult, spoke of his forced foray into boy scouts. Unaware of his diagnosis and extremely concerned about their son's increased social withdrawal, Kent's parents enrolled him at the age of seventeen into the boy scouts. They threatened to not help pay for college if he didn't actively participate and go on at least two camping trips. Because he didn't have any merit badges, the head scout leader placed him in a troop composed mostly of middle school children. Miserable, he huddled in the corner during the meetings, refusing to talk with anyone. Two painful months later, his parents recognized that this wasn't an appropriate socialization forum for Kent and he quickly left the group. More effective ways of easing your child into a more social arena are with music and art lessons in which there is a smaller emphasis on socializing and a greater emphasis on the activity. As many of my AS adult patients have told me, it takes one to two months for an AS child or adult to warm up to a situation. If, as a parent, you feel you need more specific direction, there are social therapists who can help guide the parents and child to better cope with normal childhood experiences that may be overwhelming to the overly sensitive Asperger child.

Teenage Years

Somewhere around puberty, the AS child takes a giant step backward. First, there is the social maturity delay. The child with AS is a few years socially delayed.

If you think of the AS teenager as sixteen going on twelve, it will give you a better sense of their emotional maturity. Paradoxically, their intellectual maturity may be much higher than their chronological age, which can lead to some strange interactions.

> Sarah, an AS student in her first week of college, visited her guidance counselor. He discussed her academic achievement and where she would best fit in. Impressed with her attentive and mature demeanor during the discussion, he remarked, "You seem quite mature compared to the average freshman student." Puzzled by this harmless remark, and not sure whether this was a compliment or an insult, Sarah said in an assertive way, "What do you mean?" The counselor was astounded by this rapid change of attitude and quickly remarked as he directed her to the door, "You don't have acne." Sarah didn't understand the counselor was complimenting her in this rhetorical question.

The AS teen is also amazingly gullible. This is often a source of amusement for their peers as the new AS teen will pretty much believe anything told to them. It can also be a source of trouble. A fourteen-year-old AS teenager and her older sister were crossing a busy street. There was an eighteen-wheeler truck with a ground clearance of five feet. Some young men urged the girl to walk under the truck. Fortunately, her older sister stopped her just in time as the light turned green and the truck drove away. Later, as the older sister asked her younger AS sister why she would even think of doing such a thing, the girl said that the men in the car suggested it. It just never dawned on her that other people would steer her into doing something potentially harmful.

The AS teenager thinks literally and therefore rarely understands jokes. As the non-AS teenager is starting to get interested in the opposite sex and status, the AS teen is still back with preteen interests and values. There is little interest in AS teenager girls in make-up, or flirting, or flexing muscles, or sex in guys. Clothing is still something to protect the person from the elements rather than making a social statement. While puberty is difficult for any child, for the AS child, it is extremely confusing. Why aren't the other children still interested in Nintendo or riding bikes? Often the AS child only had one or two early childhood friends, now those friends even seem to reject him. To make matters worse, most AS children tend to be awkward and rarely do well in sports. And while these observations are often the norm, there are exceptions. Some AS children are social or wear fashionable clothing and may even have these as their special interests topics. But in my experience, they are very much in the minority. Puberty is when the AS angst seems more prominent.

Confusion about Sex

Kelly, a gentle AS twelve-year-old boy, had been friendly with Ellen for several years at school. Excited about an upcoming dance, Kelly asked

Ellen to go. Confused by Ellen's rejection and without realizing that it was inappropriate, Kelly went to talk it over with her. Each time she made an excuse that she couldn't talk just then. Again not realizing that she was clearly uncomfortable with his desire to talk with her, Kelly persisted. Finally, Ellen accused him of stalking her and went to the school authorities. Fortunately, when Kelly's parents' found out, they had a long talk with him. Even though it was still puzzling to him, Kelly trusted his parents' judgment and stopped trying to talk with Ellen. Two months later, they resumed their pre-dance friendly relationship.

Social Rules

There is no tactful way to put this. AS teens are dense socially. While they can be trained to follow social rules, they will never understand their purpose. By nature, AS people are direct and don't understand the nuances of the teenage years. The concept of flirting is alien. One AS teen was asked out by the captain of the junior varsity basketball team in high school. Wanting to be normal but quite unprepared for what this meant, the relationship lasted all of one day. Comfortably reading in the library, she couldn't understand what all the fuss was about when she said she would pass on eating lunch with him to finish the book. Fortunately, the subsequent "break-up" was not particularly traumatic as it made very little difference to her whether she was involved in this relationship or not.

Depression

In some AS children, depression appears around puberty as the teenager becomes increasingly aware of just how different they are from the non-AS teen. Sometimes, with good role modeling, this is a transient stage and the AS teen accepts the difference and plays to its strengths. With others, this is when the teen turns to drug use and drinking to help her fit in starts. The anxious look of early childhood may be replaced by a sulky, angry, or defensive look. Others will resist any attempts to learn normal social behaviors and become loners. They retreat into their special interests and use this as the parameter for dealing with the world. This is often the time of intense computer gaming especially in role-playing games. In these fantasy communities, the other people in the game can't see the unusual mannerisms. In some cases, the AS teen will step into this world and pretty much step out of their own world. They will finish high school and "move" into the basement and play for days at a time. In situations like this, therapists can intervene effectively.

In too many AS teens, negative self-talk becomes the norm. Their ever-increasing awareness of their lack of social awareness and the paucity of support and encouragement for their strengths can lead to repeated pejorative comments such as, "I'm crazy" or "I'm a lunatic."

In AS, depression is additionally difficult to treat as there is often a difficulty in explaining one's feelings. Some attempt to explain their feelings by talking within the context of their topic of interest. One teenage son, fixated on the Civil War, would explain his feelings to his parents based on Civil War battles. This would frustrate his parents as unless they studied the Civil War battles, they would have no idea what he was trying to say. All efforts to encourage him to talk about his own feelings went unheeded. Civil War was his comfort zone when he felt under attack. Later, after years of fruitless attempts to understand, his parents learned that he could discuss his feelings if given time and a nonthreatening environment. They learned they would lose every head-on argument, but they were infinitely more effective if they sat down and talked in a nonjudgmental way.

As the teenager descends into depression, he will often get labeled oppositional defiant disorder (ODD). While many dispute the existence of such a condition, no one disputes the behavior. These teenagers put up a wall of rejection to most suggestions given by any authority figure. They are often argumentative, disruptive, tend to swear, and in general are fairly unpleasant to be around. These teens are extremely hard to reach. First, they generally refuse to go to a therapist to discuss what is going on; and second, their parents are exhausted, not sure what to do and tend to give up. If you realize that underneath the hard exterior is a confused, hurt, and fearful person, you can sometimes reach them. By this point, the AS child and teenager is exquisitely sensitive to criticisms or reprimands as that is often what most of them have been hearing for years. There is no good or easy advice to a parent at this stage. Without wishing to cast blame, I find that parents who are overwhelmed in their own life, often from circumstances beyond their control like divorce or illness, tend to have the children with these behaviors. I would suggest that you settle your own life first and then when you are stronger reach out to your teenager. In most cases, removing your child from the house should be a last resort. The group homes for troubled children may not even know AS exists, much less how to work with a person with this condition. And once AS teenagers are thrust in among harder, often mentally or emotionally disturbed peers, they are either bullied or they pick up new harmful behaviors. Some conventional medicine may make the behavior less extreme, but the only medicine I have seen really help without dulling the child is classical homeopathy. Often after the correct homeopathic remedy, they will be more receptive to parents, teachers, and counselors. I'll discuss the use of homeopathy with AS in great depth in Chapter 10.

MAKING POOR DECISIONS

There are several specific concerns relating to AS about this. First, because of the poor social skills, the AS teen will latch onto a group of kids who may be engaging in illegal activity. Always the gullible one, the AS child may be the fall guy and end up in jail. In one case, a group of teenagers told the AS teen that they would be right out after getting a few things from a convenience store. About five minutes later, they came running out of the convenience store to the sound of police sirens. Confused as to what was going on, the AS teen froze and was quickly apprehended. When an AS child or adult is put into a confrontational state, one of two things most often occurs: they will either shut down or become aggressive. In this case, the teenager shut down and couldn't remember either his contact information or those of his "friends." It looked like defiance and complicity with the theft, when in reality, at that moment, he wouldn't have been able to communicate the most simple of information. With no other suspects available, this AS teen was charged with theft. In reality, the only two things he was guilty of was making a poor choice of friends and being extremely naive.

THE ASPERGER SYNDROME NERD

With a lot of support from the parents, there is also the well-adjusted AS nerd. This teenager accepts his social sideline place at school and devotes himself toward his special interests and grades. With fewer distractions, he excels in both. You find many of these children in boy scouts and similar organizations. They adhere to the rules and do well in this structured environment. They are still rigid in personality, but they have figured out how to adapt to the unspoken rules of the general society. These kids tend to go on to become scientists, engineers, or college professors. They do well and often don't even know they have AS. They just attribute their behavior to being like Dad or Mom.

ADVICE TO PARENTS

One of my biggest concerns as a physician treating AS is the parental rejection or conversely the indulgence that can occur. I'm hoping by now, you are seeing that AS characteristics can be passed from generation to generation. However, when either parent distances themselves from a child, the child feels defective. Many AS adults will recall being treated as if incapable despite evidence of clear intelligence. The AS child must be allowed to grow up. It does take a considerable amount of time and effort on the parents' part to help the child with this transition. Simple things that other children will pick up easily must be explained and then re-explained, multiple times. In some ways, it's like a person learning the English language. English is full of contradictions. We learn rules and then we learn to break them in certain circumstances. As I tell the parents of AS children over and over again, the time and effort you put into your child to help them grow will result in a successful, confident, and productive adult. This process will be long, difficult, and frustrating, and require even more patience than you think you have. Often the gains are sporadic and not in the order you are expecting. For example, with one patient, the parents were completely focused on his chewing on his clothing. At each visit, they discussed the chewing despite the fact that over the three months, according to the parents, the child's outbursts had decreased by 90 percent, his anxiety was down significantly, and he no longer had stomachaches every day. The parents focused on the chewing as that was the most embarrassing aspect of AS to them. Fortunately, they understood when I talked to them about not becoming fixated on one aspect and continue to look at the big picture. With the pressure off the chewing, this behavior stopped a month later. Think of how hard we, as adults, work on various goals such as building our own businesses or getting an education to support our families. Even if we have an economic downturn or do poorly on a test, we keep our goal in mind and keep working. We need to adopt this attitude with AS children. How much more important are the stakes when we realize what these children's futures will be like if we don't put in this effort.

In some parents, I see a driving need to make their AS children "normal." If your child has AS, his or her brain is wired differently. He or she will never be "normal." They may learn to adapt to social rules and tone down their behavior, but they will always have a bit more anxiety and overreactivity than others. If your child is happy and his or her behavior is not harming herself or anyone else, then give the child latitude. Often AS adults don't have fond memories of high school. One AS middle-aged man had a positive experience. Every day at lunchtime, he quickly ate his lunch and retreated to a favorite chair in the school library. He looked forward to that half-hour of delving into all sorts of scientific books. Looking back, he realized that this was when there was no stimuli bombarding him and he could relax his nervous system. It wasn't relaxing to him to eat lunch with others with the strain of small talk. Eating lunch with others was just one more class in his day. Once his parents found out, they were concerned. Fortunately, they say that he was happy and interacted well with other students during class. He just needed downtime to recuperate. When I discussed this situation with a high school administrator, she said that if the school had realized this, they would have discouraged it. She was rethinking school policy about the extent they were working to have AS children conform to behaviors of non-AS students. Think what is in the best interest of your child. Are they happy and doing well academically? Do they have a healthy self-esteem? If so, trust them to make sound decisions. When this teenager tried not going to the library, he found himself increasingly agitated in the afternoon. Not everyone needs to be alike.

Along with wondering how much latitude to give AS students, there is a confusion about whose job it is to help them. I have listened to dozens of parents and half as many school personnel discuss the confrontational situation that occurs in many school settings over whose responsibility it is to give primary support to these children. Of course, the answer is that they both play an important role. But ultimately, the child is the product of his parents and they have the primary responsibility. They need to learn as many techniques from school personnel including occupational therapists and follow through with the same exercises at home. Raising an AS child is time-consuming. Successful adults report that in their childhood at least one parent spent one to two hours each evening helping them with assignments and processing the school experience. On the weekends, the parents spent even more time working on activities to build their children's self-confidence. Successful AS adults frequently credit their success to their parents' efforts and never-failing confidence in them.

It's sad to see young AS adults living at home or not driving a car because of the parents' fear and incomplete guidance. AS children are not defective—their brains are just wired a bit differently. One adult commented on his childhood this way: "My parents thought my flat voice meant that I was mentally deficient. They didn't push me academically like they did my siblings. It wasn't until I graduated from high school and was accepted at several colleges did they start to painstakingly slowly change this perception of me." There is an important balance to be met between coddling the child and rejection. Either extreme leads to problems. The parent who fiercely defends and isolates the AS child from others in hopes of protecting him from the world is doing the child a great disservice. That AS child will grow up and be poorly prepared for adulthood that is predominantly not AS. But, please don't take this as an endorsement of the "tough love" mentality. Bullying an AS child with repeated phrases such as "grow up," "be a man," or "act normal," isn't productive or effective. Kent's forced participation in boy scouts didn't help him as it was an inappropriate forum for his age and ability. Every child must be allowed to fall when learning to walk. The AS child is no different. But when a child stumbles, brush them off, guide them through the pitfalls, and let them try again. It took one teen three tries to get his driver's license because of his test anxiety. He then followed it by an accident-free record of more than twenty years. Another practiced in a deserted parking lot on weekends for three months before deciding she was ready to go on the road. As her father put it, "It may have taken her longer than my other children, but she knew when she was ready." Interestingly enough, this father feels safer when his AS daughter is driving than with anyone else. She stays focused on the rules of the road and is an extremely defensive driver. Instead of projecting a sense of incompetence onto the AS, work on building self-esteem. Understand that there is a different timetable with the AS child.

One father counseled his AS daughter by saying, "We may be different, but it's our job to fit into their world." With these few words the father acknowledged his similarities to his daughter and gently pushed her to work on getting skills to help her better cope with the world. This gentle extension of the AS child's boundaries is critical for her development.

Because of the lack of social skills and peculiar mannerisms, AS children can be embarrassing. Well-meaning friends and family will offer often unwanted counsel on just how to raise these kids. Strangers will often chime in with harsh words or stares. The always-present assumption is that if the parents just did a better job, the child would be normal. It's hard to stay compassionate with a child who is shrieking at someone touching him or who has just had an embarrassing meltdown in the supermarket or mall because of a sensory overload. But if you put it in perspective it may ease this pressure.

Amy was a model mother of a wonderful AS son. She wanted to do everything just right. But despite her best efforts, Brian, like any other child, responded well to some things and not to others. He attended regular school classes, but was fairly shy. She redoubled her efforts to "make him normal" and was feeling frustrated when a misfortune changed her perspective. One of her sister's very healthy and normal children was in a car accident. This happy, bouncy little girl was now in a wheel chair. When I hadn't got her biweekly check-in, I gave her a call. She told me about her niece. She reflected "Once you put things in perspective, Brian is a happy child and is doing great!" She decreased the pressure both off herself and her son.

Because of their naiveté and innocence, AS children are captivating. Once you get to know them and look past the quirky behavior, they are funny, sweet, and really want to do the right thing. Some conformity is needed to adapt in our society. But when we try to make them conform to an unnecessary degree, we are breaking their spirits. Is it really important if your child has one friend versus ten, goes to the prom, or achieves whatever social milestone you have set out for them? If given their own head, the AS child will often far exceed expectations in academics and real achievements. Instead, we need to gently but firmly guide them with compassion. In many ways, compassion, love, patience, and perseverance are our strongest tools in helping these children lead a productive and happy life. When we use these tools, we are also giving children a means for conducting the rest of their lives. Treat this condition as you would any other medical condition. Get expert advice and then figure out what is best for your particular situation. All the extreme behaviors discussed in this chapter were before treating these children with natural medicine. After these treatments, these behaviors and thought patterns were dramatically improved. The key is to start when your child is young when her self-esteem is intact. It is much harder to get a young adult to make these changes. And while natural medicine will never take the place of good, loving, parenting, it will make the job easier.

What I have seen in my practice reflects the rest of the population; the person's childhood environment affects their future. I consistently find that the AS children who are nurtured, encouraged, and accepted do well. Instead of punishing social and behavioral differences, the parents and schools reward their strengths and teach them more appropriate social skills. When this doesn't happen, the child feels rejected and defective. This negative self-image often persists into adulthood. In fact, an adult with AS said, "Having Asperger Syndrome is like being raised in one universe only to find that you were born and are more suited to living in a parallel universe."

CHAPTER 3

What Asperger Syndrome Looks Like in an Adult

The typical Asperger adult replaces the confusion of adolescence with adaptive behavior that tends to work most of the time. While he retains many of the same characteristics, he has learned to temper them. Depending on the stability of his childhood, he may never realize that his anxiety and lack of social skills could be perceived as a problem. He goes on to have a job, a family, and socializes within the context of his special interests. In fact, many adults with Asperger Syndrome (AS) have no idea that they have this condition. They may consider themselves not particularly social, somewhat anxious, and limited in interests outside a very narrow range of subjects. They may even admit that others find them quirky, but since they have carved out a simple life, they are often content. In fact, it's only when their children have been diagnosed that they begin to consider the diagnosis for themselves. Their behavior isn't as dramatic as their child's but it has the same basic characteristics. Often, the condition is moderated in adulthood by compensatory behavior learned in childhood. The person masks the anxiety and says little or simply withdraws in social situations. They describe themselves as reserved, while others might call them a bit peculiar and odd. Temple Grandin, a well-known speaker and author on the autism spectrum talks about the "happy Asperger adult." There are large numbers of AS adults holding down steady jobs in the technology, academic, and scientific communities, as did their parents before them.

For others with AS, it was virtually impossible to not be aware of the differences. They often had either more severe cases or seriously dysfunctional childhoods. If not given the tools to adapt in childhood, they either continue to live with their parents in their adulthood or in a government-funded assisted living situation. Often there are problems with anger resulting in outbursts and overreactions. There may be concurrent diagnoses such as Asperger and bipolar disorder or borderline personality disorder.

Despite the differences in the functional levels of AS adults, there are many characteristics that all share in work, friendship, marriage, and family. When you read this chapter, please keep in mind that AS is a continuum of mild to severe cases. I've tried to include a wide spectrum of behaviors that will give a better sense of the adult AS thought pattern. You may see yourself, your adult child, or your significant other in some of the descriptions, but not all.

THE WORK PLACE

In the workplace, if managed effectively, AS adults make excellent steadfast employees. They tend to be single-minded about their jobs and are happy to delve into minutiae. Tony Attwood, arguably one of the world's best authorities on AS, says that for most adults with AS, their job is an extension of themselves and that losing that job is like losing their soul. The typical AS adult is frequently happiest and most productive in semisolitary jobs such as research positions, night shift employees, and solo entrepreneurs. Many large technical corporations employ adults with AS. Temple Grandin, a very successful, high-functioning autistic technical designer, has joked that NASA is an institution for autistic adults.

If working for a large corporation, the AS employee does best if given a project and then allowed to proceed on his own. One computer engineer would be given a task and would literally sit at his desk staring into space for two to three days and then write the entire program from start to finish. Initially, he hid the staring by pretending to read related technical books; but eventually his employer realized what was happening and accepted his unusual but extremely productive work style. His turnaround time on a project was considerably faster than his peers. If this engineer was disturbed during this two to three-day development phase, he would be stymied and would have to start the process all over again. He worked in this manner for years until a new boss took over. Unable to adapt to an inflexible supervisor, he quit.

The AS employee is so dedicated to his work that it becomes an extension of himself. He will spend many extra hours, even to the detriment of his marriage, completing the given task. Despite and conversely because of this strong work ethic, the AS employee often alienates coworkers and bosses with her abrupt and less than diplomatic manner. AS adults often have difficulty with tact and patience and, in some cases, have a tendency to overreact. In other cases, they aren't even aware that their response is extreme. In their minds, they are simply sharing their point of view. They don't necessarily register the recipients' response to their statements and are often genuinely puzzled and shocked to find that they have hurt others' feelings. One engineer so alienated his boss and coworker that his boss remarked, "You are the best engineer I've ever hired. If I could keep you isolated in a room and just slide the projects under the door, you would have a job forever." Sadly, this really talented man couldn't hold on to this or any other job and ended up having dozens of jobs in the same amount of years. A Wall Street journal article clearly demonstrates this dilemma. It describes multiple adults on the spectrum who, despite a college education, have difficulty in keeping their jobs. In one case, a successful relative stepped in, hired the person for a year and taught them sufficient social skills for them to go back to their own field and succeed.[1] Perhaps the best advise is for parents to step in and groom the child about social skills or for the adult to hire a coach or therapist skilled in working with adults with AS and learn them.

A related trait to many AS employees is that they often don't participate in office social interactions and usually make no effort to keep up with subjects like sports or movies that might help them better with small talk. Instead, they prefer to work. If invited to lunch, they will discuss work. Which means, they are often invited once, but not again. Similarly, they don't understand office politics. The person with AS may have trouble understanding why interpersonal dynamics plays such a dominant role in the workplace. One young AS in-house insurance adjuster, working with over a hundred other women, welcomed the lunch break as a time to retreat from her coworkers, rather than socialize. As was to be expected, this seemed very strange to the others. She didn't understand how this might have contributed to her being passed over for promotion despite very favorable reviews. A young man working in a warehouse performed his job well, but seemed completely unable to resolve conflicts with his coworkers. He confused being assertive with being abrasive. This is a common theme. There is often an all or nothing mentality in the AS population. They can be extremely passive, resulting in being bullied by their coworkers. In some ways this is a continuation of the bullying that commonly happens in the AS childhood. In an extreme case, one worker was physically abused by one of her coworkers. It wasn't until another coworker witnessed the incident that the abuse was identified and stopped. But when trying to change this, they can overreach their goal and become aggressive.

Because of the huge deficit of communication skills, the AS adult is frequently misunderstood. A talented engineer received a harassment disciplinary action when he admonished a fellow worker about recycling. Thinking he was simply being proactive, he unwittingly scared the other person with his intensity. The AS person can be painfully naïve and completely shocked that to them a simple miscommunication would be received as a threat. This behavior, simply reflecting a lack of social skills, led to a fairly widespread ostracism.

The emotional shutdown in the child following a reprimand manifests similarly in the adult.

Brian is a successful part-time instructor at a college. Generally well-liked by his students because of his passion for the subject, he routinely received very positive reviews. Therefore, he was quite surprised to be called in by the Dean and given a gentle reprimand for a student's comment. As if his brain froze, he tried to defend himself but could not remember the names of *any* of his students or the particulars of this complaint. His mind went completely blank. Stumbling, he admitted to being completely confused by this and could provide no adequate explanation. The meeting concluded with the Dean sternly advising him to adjust his behavior. Brian left the office and attempted to compose himself. Within a few minutes, his mind cleared and he could remember the specific circumstance and the student involved and realized that there was a simple miscommunication. The complaint wasn't directed against him, but against school policy. The student was using a forum that she knew would be read to relay her message. Armed with this information, he returned to the Dean only to be told that the matter was settled.

This brain freeze when reprimanded can lead to some extreme adaptive behavior. Some people with AS go to great lengths to avoid reprimands or confrontations. They become almost perfectionistic in order to not have any negative attention drawn to their work. Interestingly enough, this brain freeze doesn't seem to occur when the confrontation is between business peers or when the AS person is in the supervisory position.

Even though the AS person tends to need much less social interaction than others, that is not to say that he needs none. The problem is, the AS person often has trouble distinguishing between a friend and friendly behavior. She may glum onto the one coworker who says "Hi" to her in the morning, especially when she is virtually ignored by the others. In her mind, this simple greeting constitutes a friendship; while in the other person's mind they are merely work acquaintances. This can lead to confusion. Fortunately, AS people have a radar for other AS people and in large corporations can usually find a kindred spirit.

As an extension of their ability to understand office politics, the AS employees make poor team project members. They can easily get frustrated with the politics, small talk, and perceived inefficiency within the group. They often can't effectively articulate their thoughts verbally and may appear confused. This is extremely misleading as, if given the chance to put their thoughts in writing, they often astound the group with their clarity of thought. It is extremely common for people on the autism spectrum to communicate better in writing than verbally. Possibly as a result of this deficiency in verbal communication, they can prefer getting and completing an assignment versus being dependent on others to complete their portions on time and up to the standard.

In addition to the lack of social skills, many AS employees may have sensory issues that can affect their job performance. Sensory issues may range from reactions to the fluorescent lights overhead to the abrasive voice of the person in the next cubical. For the AS employee, these issues can be debilitating. For example, an abrasive voice for most people is just that abrasive. For someone with sensory issues, the voice might actually hurt the person's ears. Imagine someone scraping a blackboard over and over in the cubical next to you. One AS employee wore a hat and earplugs at work. She was remarkably productive, so this odd behavior was ignored by her supervisor. Another light-sensitive employee wore sunglasses. The sensory issues may lead to increased overreactivity and decreased ability to concentrate. Some employers will allow full spectrum desk lights or will disconnect the fluorescent lights directly above the workstation. Others are less accommodating. Some people who have been diagnosed with AS turn to the Americans with Disabilities Act of 1990 to resolve disputes in the workplace. This act guarantees that the employer makes a reasonable effort to accommodate the employee's disability. There are benefits and liabilities to this Act. By invoking it, you are inviting your employer to regard you as "disabled." This may dramatically affect your ability to advance. Essentially, you will win the battle but lose the war. However, in some circumstances, where the job is not a career but a livelihood, this may be the correct action. It's best to take time and analyze the cost and benefit of using this law.

THE ASPERGER MIDDLE-AGE BURNOUT

There is a curious phenomenon that seems to hit the middle-age person with AS; they start to have trouble coping on their previous level. Working with AS support groups, I see middle-aged members, previously able to function in the workplace no longer able to work and ending up on disability. For example, men who had government jobs and had been the primary breadwinners for years, being fired or let go at work and unable to regroup and hunt for a new job. I was wondering aloud about this over a luncheon with a psychologist colleague of mine, Dr. Leslie Carter, who treats the same population. She had noted this same behavior and attributed it to adrenal exhaustion from years of pumping out high levels of epinephrine from prolonged severe anxiety. Not only were these AS people dealing with their regular levels of anxiety, but they were also working extremely hard to maintain a façade of normalcy. Some AS people seemed to slip through this burnout crack. The common denominator was diet and relaxation. Those who ate an excellent diet with no sugar and who had some regular form of relaxation such as meditation or yoga, naturally supported and replenished their adrenal glands and avoided the burnout.

FRIENDSHIPS

The AS person often doesn't have the same need for friendships as the average person does. In fact, and especially in men, the issue of friendship may not even emerge if the person is employed and married. The casual acquaintances at work and the single friendship with their spouse are often sufficient. When they do have friends, the friendship will appear considerably different from a conventional one. The AS friendship is often based on function rather than socialization. For example, the AS person will want to get together for a purpose such as hiking or biking rather than to socialize at a baby shower or shopping. During breaks, they may discuss biking equipment or different hiking paths rather than share personal information or more general small talk. If the other party unwittingly initiates a conversation on a charged subject for the AS person, the AS person will respond with a flood of information delivered in a forceful, unrelenting manner. All attempts to change the subject will be ignored until the discourse is over. Of course, some people with AS are able to control this, but not all. The intensity of the AS person is not conducive to frequent visits—a welcome relief on both sides. The AS person is drained from having to maintain a normal façade for any length of time. However, if the AS person can get past the anxiety, they can become a loyal and steadfast friend. As one non-AS woman said of her AS friend, "When we get together, there is no small talk, only honest talk. She is direct and real. I never have to wonder if she is telling me what I want to hear." Living only five miles apart, this friendship has lasted for years. They have never gone shopping or to a movie or any other form of socialization. They simply get together for tea or lunch every other month. The friend routinely gives presents and Christmas cards; while her AS friend does neither. After the AS friend explained the anxiety level in trying to pick out an appropriate gift, her friend suggested she just forego the formalities. Often AS people will link up with other mildly dysfunctional people sharing some of the same characteristics. For example, a person with AS may become friends with someone with OCD (obsessive-compulsive disorder) or depression. The AS person is often remarkably tolerant. You may see this in high school or college campuses. Two quirky kids becoming friends because they were both on the social fringe only to revel in how similarly they thought. One AS home-schooling mom became quick friends with another woman who seemed to have similar traits. Ten years later, they realized why after their children were diagnosed with AS. An AS man stayed friends with a former non-AS coworker for almost thirty years. They discovered that they could only tolerate each other's company for short periods of time, but that they enjoyed each other's correspondence very much. Occasionally, you will find a very social AS person, but this is less common.

One of the biggest social challenges to the AS adult is what they perceive as personality inconsistencies in others. For the AS person, getting invited to a bar or out to dinner by coworkers, can be a disturbing experience. They perceive the usually predictable and steady coworker as changing their personality when they leave work or drink alcohol. This is baffling to the person with AS as no such change takes place with them. They don't have a work versus personal persona. And it can be disconcerting to them to witness this transformation in others. What others may perceive as normal adult conversation, including sexual innuendoes or jokes, may make the AS person extremely uncomfortable. Control and consistency help stabilize the AS person. Even something as basic as watching a sitcom together may lead to intense stress for the AS person. The AS person often doesn't get or appreciate the standard broad humor on television. They may get indignant over what they perceive as injustices to one of the characters. TV antics are not regarded as funny but as hurtful. This failure to see what others perceive as humor pervades everyday conversations. Unlike the child who just didn't comprehend the joke, the adult with AS comprehends the joke but just doesn't understand how it is funny, because to them it isn't. They may laugh if others laugh following the joke or they simply ignore it. The other person may often prompt "that was a joke."

Finally, and perhaps most damaging to maintaining a friendship is initiation. The AS person will rarely initiate an activity, unless extremely comfortable with the friend. This can be frustrating to the non-AS person as it can be misconstrued as a lack of interest. With some honest communication and effort, this can be overcome.

MARRIAGE

AS spouses are often amazingly loyal, devoted, and boring. They are often content with a simple life and are truly baffled by the discontent of their husband or wife. One wife spoke of her AS husband in this way: "He is devoted to me, his children and his job. He works very hard, provides well, and attends church regularly. He is honest, kind and thoughtful. And all I can think about is leaving him. He is never spontaneously affectionate except to our children when they were very young. I have never been made to feel sexy or desired or even needed." Though this theme is frequently echoed by the non-AS spouse, the AS spouse views things quite differently. He is most often very committed to the marriage, but will have confusion as to demonstrate this. He is rarely affectionately demonstrative in the conventional way, but will show his emotions in a more practical way. If the AS spouse is feeling loving, he may do the dishes or she might make a meal that the husband really enjoys. Attempts to train an AS person to be affectionate generally result in contrived gestures that are more mechanical than spontaneous. This extends into the bedroom.

While there are exceptions to every rule, most AS adults have low libidos. There doesn't appear to be a medical reason for this. However, if you consider the sensory issues, the overload of touch and smell may be possible reasons. Many adults have mentioned extremely cold hands and feet due to anxiety that may further dampen their enthusiasm. Unless, they have a spouse with a comparable low libido, this can cause trouble in the marriage. It will seem as if it is a personal rejection, rather than a sensory rejection.

Additionally, the sensory issues that affect the workplace also affect the home. Without the pressure of a paycheck at home forcing adaptation, AS adults often avoid sensory overload by simply not putting themselves in that situation. An adult can stay home on the Fourth of July or simply not go to movie theatres or music concerts. The AS adult may wear very bland or similar clothes—almost like a uniform. They may need to withdraw into their rooms for long stretches. When they do talk, they tend to be self-absorbed and less concerned about others. This is different from selfishness. They don't want a lot of things for themselves. Instead they just tend to simply not consider the needs and problems of others. In psychology terminology, this is called "theory of mind." It is almost as if they aren't aware that others have needs. Once the needs are pointed out, the AS adult will respond appropriately. That means little things from helping with the children, to taking out the trash, to tidying up the living room, may need to be spelled out. For example, one husband after repairing dents in his children's room, had to ask his AS wife to discourage the children from putting more dents into the walls. Because he didn't complain, she didn't recognize it as the problem it was becoming. She was more focused on cooking, cleaning, and helping three children with their homework and extracurricular activities and simply regarded these dents as a byproduct of having rambunctious male children. Once the issue came onto her radar screen, the wall dents stopped. In another case, the wife needed to explain to her AS husband that it was normal to give her an idea of where he was taking their one car on the weekend, instead of just driving off to the hardware store without any thought of her schedule or needs for the car. While, this isn't the case in every marriage, it still affects a sizeable percentage. And again, if the AS adult had a good role model, this may not even be an issue.

As mentioned earlier, there is commonly some measure of obsessive-compulsive behavior in the AS population. The obsessive compulsive component of AS might show up as compulsive buyers in adulthood. In their one-mindedness about a subject, they might purchase dozens of books or multiple items related to the subject. One wife had a chest full of antique jewelry, while a husband had thousands of dollars of electronic gadgetry. While this immoderate spending similarly occurs with non-AS people, with this group the obsessive buying is generally confined to a single subject. More commonly, people with AS are unusually frugal and will not make new purchases even when garments or furniture are worn out, even when there is no financial strain. If given the control of the finances, an AS adult will usually do an extremely good job.

The AS spouse may have trouble with change. They don't understand natural transitions in a marriage. For example, the early stages of a marriage often include constant companionship. Frequent phone calls and trips for chores are often jointly done. This phase ends and the two people transition into a combination of solitary and shared activities within their relationship. For the person with AS, this transition is difficult and in a few cases can lead to the AS spouse virtually stalking the non-AS spouse. He will follow his wife around while she does her chores or will continue discussions long past their natural conclusion. This doesn't seem to happen as much if the AS spouse's parents had a healthy marriage and a more balanced marriage model was learned.

Another instance of stalking-like behavior is in an attempt to resolve conflicts. The AS spouse's poor communication skills are very obvious during marital arguments. They lose their train of thought and seem to revert to a purely emotional state. Sometimes that emotion is anger, but more often it is hurt. Unfortunately, the AS spouse is often so unaware of her feelings that she doesn't even realize when she is upset. One husband commented that he knew when his AS wife was upset or stressed with him before she did because she would start talking like Data of the 1990s Star Trek series. She would stop using contractions and formalized her speech. For some, it's almost as if the excessive emotion has cut off the analytical part of the brain. They stumble, are completely unable to explain their actions. And they become locked into a fixed thought pattern, which they demonstrate by resorting to repetition of the same few phrases. When the conflict stymies and the spouse withdraws, the AS spouse may follow the spouse around seeking a resolution. Needless to say, this behavior is annoying and can appear like harassment. To make matters worse, when they calm down and collect their thoughts, even if it's several hours later, they will reengage to better explain their views only to be accused of wanting to reignite a fight. This pattern can be broken, but it requires both spouses to stay calm and make an earnest effort to hear each other's points of view.

There are many other areas of miscommunication within the marriage including literalism. The non-AS spouse needs to understand that the AS spouse will take them literally. For example, after having tacos once a week for six months, a husband told his AS wife that he didn't want to have tacos anymore. Taking this literally, she stopped serving tacos for years. A few years later, her husband asked "Why don't we have tacos anymore"? Puzzled, she replied, "Don't you remember? Four years ago, you told me to stop making them." For the AS spouse, words are often set in stone. It would have been more helpful if the husband had said, "We have been having tacos a lot lately, and I'm a bit tired of them. Let's hold off on having them for several months."

Once a diagnosis is made, it often profoundly affects the stability of the marriage. I often hear stories of men who have been the primary breadwinners in the family for decades find themselves the object of patronizing behavior after the AS diagnosis was made. Suddenly, all the quirky behavior has a name. What the spouse often fails to recognize is that AS adults often partner with other affected adults. The non-AS spouse may have OCD, depression, generalized anxiety, borderline personality disorder, or AD(H)D. Some even have debilitating conditions such as fibromyalgia, which have an emotional dysfunctional component. The AS spouse will be extremely tolerant of his partner's condition; a tolerance that is not always reciprocated. One wife of an AS husband bemoaned her lot. It was extremely obvious from talking with her that she was profoundly Attention Deficit Disorder (ADD). I suggested that marital problems are rarely one-sided and that it was easy to blame difficulties on the spouse's AS diagnosis. It might be more beneficial if she was evaluated for ADD and see its effect on the marriage as well.

Another disturbing trend is family interference. In one case, a reasonably happily married couple of eight years was divorced after the wife was diagnosed with AS. His parents and siblings told him to get out before there were children. The irony was that she was the main breadwinner and had a very responsible job. The non-AS husband had bouts of depression during which his AS wife was very supportive. In this case, the AS wife became involved with another man one year after her divorce. She was open about her diagnosis and happily, it made no difference to him. While no two marital situations are identical, it makes sense to carefully consider the dynamics in the marriage before yielding to family pressure based on a lack of understanding of the condition.

PARENTHOOD

As with any group, some AS parents make excellent parents and some don't. If the AS parent had a good role model in their own childhood, they have a template on how to raise their children. If they didn't, they may immerse themselves in the subject of parenthood and become excellent, though a bit too conscientious parents. One older couple researched every food that would help their child improve his brain function. They didn't stop there; next they went on to music and then to exercise.

Some AS parents, fearful of their child suffering a similar unhappy childhood as their own, assume a tough attitude toward the child. They maintain a stern demeanor that unfortunately, worsens the situation. The AS child is confused in the school and social arena already, and having one or both parents not giving him the support he needs, compounds the problem. AS adults rarely marry other AS adults so the parenting is most often a blend of styles.

Another important consideration is the extent of the parent's AS symptoms. If the anxiety or sensory issues are extreme, then this will affect the child. More often, the parent finds a solution.

One AS mom raised her children without the prerequisite group parties or face or finger-painting. These traditional parts of childhood were well outside her sensory comfort zone. Happily none of her four children seemed to mind. Instead, they went for hikes and picnics and built elaborate castles and play structures as a family. The children, now adults, felt that the attention and love she gave them daily more than made up for the lack of these traditional events.

There is a common perception that AS adults have trouble expressing affection. And while this may be true between adults, I haven't witnessed this in any of the AS parents of young children. They demonstrate the same amount of physical contact and warmness compared to non-AS parents. There may be a physical detachment when the child becomes a teenager, but affection is then manifested in less overt ways. One AS father, no longer comfortable hugging his AS daughter, instead would go on walks in the park and just talk with her. An AS mom, similar to any other mom, would make special pancakes or their grown child's favorite cornbread. As the child grows older, the parent may limit the physical contact to sideway hugs, handshakes, or tentative pats on the back. It is not a lack of affection on the AS parent's part, but a physical discomfort with himself.

THE FAMILY

When speaking with a group of AS adults, the topic of family will emerge as a very painful subject. In a good situation, the AS adult is regarded as quirky and a bit asocial. In a bad situation, the AS adult is embarrassing to the parents and siblings and is virtually ignored or conversely, heralded forth as some defect that needs to be explained on a regular basis. The mother of a professional in the school system would routinely introduce her daughter to people as having AS. She would follow any comment the woman made with "don't mind her, she has Asperger Syndrome." Another AS adult recalled his father making frequent demeaning comments regarding his AS status despite his obvious intelligence, excellent grades, and acceptance into a good university.

After repeated attempts to discourage this announcement, he started introducing his family by their medical conditions: "Here is my sister with diabetes, my father with depression, and my mother with fibromyalgia." Mortified and angered, his family got the message. But while they stopped mentioning AS, they still blamed his behavior on "his condition."

When talking to AS adults about their birth families, they will often recall memories of sibling rejection. Part of this might be because of the resentment over the extra attention the AS child frequently received from the mother; while for others it might be the embarrassment of having an odd sibling. Often, after the diagnosis is made, siblings will distance themselves even further from the AS sibling even into their adult years. Interestingly enough, this can even occur with siblings who clearly have some AS characteristics themselves. It is as if the behavior without the diagnosis is OK, but with the diagnosis is not. The problem is compounded with the infrequent contact from the AS sibling. It's fairly rare to find an AS adult who stays in frequent contact with their siblings. It seems to stem from the difficulty in doing small talk. The person with AS simply won't have anything to say. A sister would visit her AS kid brother, who she had virtually raised, once a week. Some weeks he would sit quietly and let her talk, as he simply didn't have anything to say. Fortunately, she didn't interpret this as indifference. AS siblings may lose contact with a sibling for years and then pick up where they left off. One AS woman, with seven grown siblings with families of their own, just found the whole idea of birthday and Christmas gift-giving overwhelming. So, she did nothing. She liked her nieces and nephews and enjoyed their company at family reunions, but she simply did not acknowledge them the rest of the year.

If the AS adult had a healthy loving family in childhood, these strong attachments continue on into adulthood. The siblings are used to the quirky behavior and it is generally ignored.

THE LAST GENERATION OF AS ADULTS

Over the past twenty years, there has been a new generation of AS adults that don't fit this mold. Separated in school into specialized learning programs, they have not adapted to the mainstream. Labeled as disabled, they tend to live at the ages of thirty, or even up to forty, with their parents or with a roommate in an apartment while on disability. Those who work may ask or demand special accommodations in the workplace or at schools. They will get these considerations, but in return, be repeatedly overlooked for promotion. In many cases, the Disability Act has enabled them to win the battle but not the war. It is not clear if this generation is more profoundly affected or if the job of preparing them has been shunted from full-time parents to a few hours a week with one-on-one special education teachers. This is not to fault the many dedicated single parents raising Asperger children, but it is very difficult to prepare the child for the world while working full-time. The sad truth is that if the AS person hasn't learned to adapt in childhood, it becomes almost impossible for them to make the adjustments in adulthood. Even worse, these lower-functioning AS adults are becoming the hallmark by which the condition is defined. The higher-functioning parents and relatives of this AS generation are overlooked. Instead, the medical literature will study this less-abled group and make generalizations on this fragment of the AS adult population. For example, one of those generalizations is delusional beliefs. A 2005 article written by Abell and Hare states that delusional beliefs, specifically grandiose ideas and paranoia abound in AS adults.[2] There may be paranoia because of a failure to diagnose a condition commonly confused with AS called pyroluria. I rarely see grandiose ideation among high-functioning AS adults. Occasionally, I see it in lower-functioning people who may be using it as a coping mechanism to justify the inability to take an active role in the general society.

ASPERGER SYNDROME AND CRIMINALITY

In the past few years, the media has seized on crimes that involved criminals with AS. They focused on the small number of documented cases of criminals with AS and tried to make an association between AS and crime. This was refuted by a 2006 Welch study, which looked at the behavior of over 1,000,000 people. They could not find any direct link between AS and crime.[3] As with any other physical or psychological condition, there will be a tiny segment of the population that engage in crime. However, with AS there are two major potential causes for criminal behavior—poor communication skills and obsession with a single subject matter. Darius McCollum, fascinated with the New York train system, has been repeatedly arrested and jailed for driving buses and trains. This fascination started when he was a teenager. Some of the subway and bus drivers taught him how to drive the vehicles. Eventually, they gave him a uniform. The first time he took over driving a bus was when the driver fell ill and asked him to continue the route. He has never had an accident or caused any damage to the units. By the age of forty, he had spent over ten years in prison. Interestingly enough, until his last arrest, the court seemed oblivious to the possibility of AS. Here you have a person who received mixed messages from people and was unable to sort them out. On the one hand, he was taught to drive subways and buses by official drivers and even given a uniform, while on the other hand, he was being told that it was wrong. The kinds of crimes someone with Asperger may commit are those of fixation, such as computer hacking.

More often, people with AS are victims of crime. With their inability to communicate well with the police and their overreactivity, they often find themselves not only unable to explain the crime but acting seemingly irrational. It is hard to explain to the police that even as an adult, you were naïve enough to be conned and didn't understand that the friendly person wasn't really being friendly.

CHAPTER 4

Face Blindness and Place Blindness—Who Are You and Where Am I Going?

One of the most puzzling symptoms of Asperger Syndrome (AS) is prosopagnosia or face blindness. Just as it sounds, face blindness is the inability to recognize faces. The person can see faces perfectly clearly, but the image fades rapidly from memory when the person is out of sight. The face-blind person will remember the hair, the glasses, and maybe even the mannerisms, but not the facial features of the other person. It seems to affect about 60 percent of all adults with AS.[1] Medical researcher, Ingo Kennerknecht, assuming that prosopagnosia was rare, tested a group of 689 middle-school children and some medical personnel. He discovered that 2.4 percent of this group had some measure of face blindness.[2] This suggests that more than one person in every fifty in the general population has face blindness. The significance of face blindness is often understated in the AS community. Because AS affects social interaction, a person unable to remember a person's face would dramatically affect his ability and confidence to successfully interact with others.

Prosopagnosia seems to affect each person in varying degrees. In some, it may take three strong contacts to be able to recall the other person's face again. Just casually being introduced and talking for a minute would not be enough to register that person for someone with prosopagnosia. For others it can take nine to ten lengthy exposures to remember the other person's face. For example, one therapist with AS and prosopagnosia would spend over an hour with each client. He would just start to recognize the client after the eighth or ninth visit. And if he saw the person at the grocery store or jogging, he wouldn't have a context and would be unable to identify the client. In more severe cases, there may be an inability to remember even close family members. Tom, a middle-aged man with prosopagnosia, engaged in an animated conversation with an attractive woman sitting next to him on an airplane. It took him several minutes before he realized, based on the conversation, that this woman was his sister. An orthodontist, used to seeing over twenty-five patients daily, introduced herself to the same patient three times in the space of twenty minutes as she left and re entered the office. An AS college woman talked with a male classmate in a coffee shop for several hours one evening feeling like she had met someone special. The next day she was unable to recognize him. Fortunately for her, he was neither face-blind nor rebuffed by her appearing indifferent to him the following day. At a medical seminar, a doctor was greeted warmly by his colleague. Puzzled, the doctor asked how they knew each other. The colleague raised his eyebrows and stiffly answered that they spent twelve hours a week on a three-month clinic shift together six years earlier. While this might initially seem humorous, it's not so funny to the person with face blindness. Others perceive them as forgetful or rude. In the business setting, it looks unprofessional; in social situations, it can be difficult to explain.

Most adults and children are completely unaware that they have face blindness. They simply don't have a frame of reference to determine it. For example, if an AS father has face blindness and isn't aware of the condition, he wouldn't look for it in his children. Also, similar to AS, it can affect several family members in varying degrees. In one family, the AS mother was severely impacted by face blindness while her non-AS children were affected to a much smaller degree and her AS daughter, not affected at all. There isn't a consistent pattern to the condition. Like color blindness, it's hard to imagine that others can see what you can't. One middle-aged woman was surprised that other people could close their eyes and picture their loved ones in their minds. Some, when they find out, take it in their stride as just another AS symptom. For others, it can be traumatizing to realize that a very fundamental part of a person's life, the ability to recognize others, especially loved ones, just doesn't work correctly. It seems that when this piece of the AS puzzle is recognized, then it explains many earlier occurrences such as lost sales jobs, friends, and social rebuffs. It definitely contributes to the sense of alienation that hallmarks the AS condition.

CHILDREN AND FACE PROSOPAGNOSIA

Face blindness is even harder to discern in children with AS because it looks like just another anxiety issue. The parent will prod the child forward and say, "Go play with Rob," not realizing that the child has no idea which little boy is Rob. Worse, he has already figured out that you can't just go up to someone and say, "Are you Rob?" So he blusters his way through and makes many mistakes. Often these kids just wander in the playground. That's not to say that an AS child wandering in the playground is always doing that because of face blindness, but it is one reason. An AS adult, in disbelief for days after being diagnosed with prosopagnosia, began to see the huge impact this condition had on her childhood. She now understood why she never had any friends in school. Sure, her military family moved a lot, but in hindsight she remembered it being really hard to tell the kids apart and then after the fourth school in four years, she just decided it wasn't worth the effort and withdrew socially. She also realized her siblings didn't seem to have this trouble.

A child with AS won't be able to tell which medium-height, plump, brown-haired woman is his teacher or the school principal. Often, the only friends the children with prosopagnosia will have will be physically distinct. One adult remembered having a short black-haired friend with glasses, while another had a tall significantly overweight child as a friend. While the child will have no frame of reference to even realize there is a problem, there might be signs that some sort of dysfunction exists. One child with AS, excited to be on his first vacation with only his grandparents, became increasingly anxious the farther he went from his home. His grandparents were surprised as this was a resilient little boy but figured that it was a case of homesickness. Finally, the child blurted out that he wasn't missing his parents, but he just couldn't remember what they looked like and that frightened him. Parents and teachers should consider face blindness if the child with AS seems almost confused, not just awkward socially. And while some children with face blindness will have some ability to see faces in their minds, all will have trouble consistently recognizing people's faces. Look for clues. The child may seem uncertain until the other person speaks or does some sort of familiar action to identify him.

TRYING TO EXPLAIN FACE BLINDNESS

Frequently, attempts to explain face blindness are met with disbelief or dismissal. Often the person with prosopagnosia will hear someone say, "I'm bad with names, too." The difference is, a person who just can't remember names will still know that they are talking to a friend or business associate, the person with prosopagnosia will feel as if they are conversing with a total stranger. When asked the color of her husband's eyes, one AS woman who had been married for seven years could not remember. The part of her brain that would pick up that detail just didn't work. Another woman, a first-time mom, was unable to identify her newborn baby in the hospital nursery. Shaken, but determined to see her baby, she surreptitiously checked the names on the various cribs. Prosopagnosia isn't a simple memory lapse, it's a memory disconnect.

Even when they discover that they have face blindness, most people are reluctant to admit it. In fact, if the AS person with face blindness decides to reveal this, she can feel very vulnerable. A young woman was attacked on campus and unable to identify her attacker except by hair and build, which was too general a description to help the police. In another case, a young boy was harassed by several classmates, but was unable to later identify these bullies. Since most police departments are unfamiliar with face blindness, the victim loses credibility very quickly. Most people with AS could remember voices, mannerisms, and hair, but would fail completely to identify the alleged perpetrator at a police lineup.

Because most people who have prosopagnosia often don't realize it, we have devised a questionnaire that might suggest whether you or your child has prosopagnosia. If you have prosopagnosia, when you read these questions, you will think, everyone has these problems. You may not even be aware you are compensating for these problems. Everyone might have some of these problems on a rare instance, but not regularly.

PROSOPAGNOSIA QUESTIONNAIRE

1. When I close my eyes, I can't clearly "see" the face of the loved one in my mind.
2. I can spend an hour or so talking to a person and not recognize them the next day.
3. I can meet someone and not recognize them fifteen minutes later.
4. I have trouble recalling who my waiter/waitress is at a restaurant.
5. I have trouble recognizing someone when they change their hairstyle (e.g., shaved a beard, cut their hair, or grow it out).
6. When starting a new job, I seem to take longer than others remembering who my coworkers are.
7. I meet people who seem to know me, but I don't know them.
8. Sometimes, I have trouble recognizing family, friends, and coworkers.
9. I greet people I think I recognize only to find out they don't know me.
10. Same-sex characters in the same general age category in a movie tend to look alike to me.
11. Others joke that I have a terrible memory for faces.
12. I can easily identify a person by their walk before they are close enough to identify by face.
13. I have a good ear for voices.
14. I tend not to use names when greeting others after they greet me, because I'm not always sure who they are.
15. I rely on a friend who is really good at remembering people when in social situations.
16. I find myself identifying people by context rather than facial characteristics. (That stocky person walking toward me must be John because I'm at work and John is a stocky man who works here.)
17. I'm not sure I would be able to recognize my sister or brother who I haven't seen in a year or two if I saw her or him on the street.
18. My child rarely identifies children at school by name.
19. My child seems confused (as well as shy) around other children.
20. Others in my family have difficulty remembering or recognizing faces.

If you answered "yes" to eight or more of these questions, then you may have face blindness and may want to have it formally tested and diagnosed.

TESTING FOR PROSOPAGNOSIA

For several decades, prosopagnosia has been generally diagnosed with tests such as the Benton Facial Recognition Test (BFRT), the Warrington Recognition

Memory for (WRMFT) Faces Test and informal testing with photographs of contemporary celebrities and political figures that would be age and culture-appropriate for the test subject. The BFRT tests the ability of subjects to recognize faces from different angles and with different shadowing. The WRMFT determines the short-term memory of a subject for faces with varying facial expressions. While these tests may give an indication of the condition, they might not take into consideration either how the person with prosopagnosia compensates or the various degrees of face blindness. For example, some people with prosopagnosia can remember faces for a minute or two. If the same face is flashed before them in those same two minutes, they will be able to identify it and therefore will not be recognized as having face blindness. Also, unless the test is timed, the person with prosopagnosia might be able to determine the identity after eight to ten seconds, which is considerably longer than the one or two seconds that most people would take in typical business or social interactions. In some instances the target face is present simultaneously with the pictures in question, allowing the test subject to determine the correct answer by comparing facial features. People with face blindness often inadvertently compensate by recognizing hairstyles and jewelry. They could easily identify the woman with fish earrings even if she looked similar to the woman with gold hoop earrings.

In an effort to make a more accurate test that would better reflect the number of people with prosopagnosia, Dr. Brad Duchaine, a researcher first from Harvard and currently with the University College in London, developed a test entitled Cambridge Face Memory Test. This test drew from the strengths from each of the earlier tests to derive a test that would more accurately diagnose people with face blindness. In this timed test, there are pictures of closely cropped faces with similar neutral expressions and lighting. The cropping avoids the test subject from recognizing hair or earrings or some alternative means. The test subject sees the targeted faces seventeen times throughout the test alongside distractor faces. While the Warrington and Benton tests are still widely used, the Cambridge Face Memory Test appears to be the most accurate test for diagnosis.

PROSOPAGNOSIA RESEARCH

Even though prosopagnosia was first identified in 1947, the scientific community has studied it more intensely in the last two decades. Prosopagnosia is generally classified into two types: trauma-induced or acquired and developmental. As its name suggests, trauma-induced prosopagnosia develops after an injury to the head. Developmental prosopagnosia (DP) is a little more complicated to explain. Because infants aren't tested for DP at birth, it's uncertain if the DP developed during gestation, early childhood, is congenital or possibly linked to another neurological condition such as AS. Most of the older scientific literature suggested that the majority of cases of prospagnosia were trauma-induced.[3, 4] More and more researchers are challenging this perception as more people without head injury are being identified as having prospagnosia. Initially, scientists thought that face blindness was caused by an injury to a specific neural pathway. But prosopagnosia, like Asperger, seems to affect each person in a slightly different way. If it were a specific neural pathway, most people with face blindness would have more similar symptoms. More importantly, if it were a specific neural pathway, it would be easier to understand and possibly to treat. But with multiple neural pathways involved, the etiology of prosopagnosia remains a mystery. J. Barton of Beth Israel Deaconess Medical Center in Boston writes, "Prosopagnosia is not a single functional disorder but a family of dysfunctions, with different patients having different degrees of impairments to various perceptual and memory stages involved in face processing."[5] Prominent prosopagnosia researchers, Bradley Duchaine from University College in London and Ken Nakayama from Harvard, similarly propose that it is a heterogeneous condition with "different cases demonstrating different types of impairments."[6]

Some researchers are analyzing autistic conditions such as Asperger Syndrome with prosopagnosia. In a 2004 article written in the medical journal *Brain*, Barton et al. ask, "Are patients with social developmental disorders prosopagnosic?"[7] He challenges the decades-old hypothesis that social dysfunction in social developmental disorders cause the face blindness. His article made several conclusions. There is no correlation between a particular autism spectrum disorder and prosopagnosia, though he did find that 66 percent of the participants with social developmental disorders such as AS had some level of face recognition difficulty. People with social impairment don't necessarily have face blindness. And in those with both social impairment and prosopagnosia, the severity of the social development did not directly correspond to the impairment of the face blindness. Marlene Behrmann of the Carnegie Mellon University concurs, "Face-processing problems are not entirely social in nature and that a visual perceptual impairment (neurological dysfunction) might also contribute."[8] Thus, having Asperger doesn't cause the face blindness. But practically speaking, face blindness definitely affects the ability to socially interact.

In an effort to better understand why face blindness occurs, researchers Galit Yovel and Nancy Kanwisher of the Massachusetts Institute of Technology used functional magnetic-resonance imaging (MRIs) to scan the brain while the person with prosopagnosia attempted to identify other people. They determined that the fusiform face area (FFA) or occipitotemporal gyrus is involved with face recognition. In trauma-induced prosopagnosia, this area is damaged. In those with developmental or hereditary prosopagnosia as would occur with up to 60 percent of those with AS, there is little sign of FFA neurological damage. Interestingly, in some but not all subjects with developmental prosopagnosia, these MRI-monitored neural responses were normal as compared to those subjects without face blindness. Again, this tells us that there are many unknown causes of prosopagnosia and that other areas besides the FFA are involved with prosopagnosia. It also gives an insight as to the varying expressions of prosopagnosia. Thomas and Martina Gruter, a geneticist team, suggest that because it often occurs in several members of the same family, it may be an autosomal dominant trait and therefore from a single gene.[9] They are trying to isolate that gene and tend to refer to developmental prosopagnosia as hereditary prosopagnosia.

More recent research questions as to whether prosopagnosia is linked to the ability to recognize facial expression. Facial expression recognition is the ability to determine the mood of the other person by looking at their facial expression. This is a completely different phenomenon than face blindness. In the AS population, this ability is frequently impaired. It's fairly common to hear the AS person not understand that others are irritated with him until the situation escalates into a confrontation. Many aren't able to recognize the narrowing eyes or furrowed brow of an irritated person, or the quiet demeanor of someone when they are sad. A 2005 article in Neurology written by Hefter et al. of Harvard Medical School found that in her test subjects, "The subjects with social developmental disorders with impaired facial identity (prosopagnosia) perceived facial expression as well as those with normal facial identity procession.[10]

Prosopagnosia Worsens Social Anxiety

In people with AS, prosopagnosia also compounds the social anxiety. Imagine meeting someone, having a wonderful stimulating conversation, and then simply not recognizing them the next day. Consider the ramifications in the workplace. If you can't remember the face of your boss, then it's necessary to find a way to compensate. To successfully navigate the business and social world, the AS person with face blindness must expend an enormous amount of energy learning to recognize others by their size, gait, hand gestures, hair, clothing style, and voice. It can be exhausting. Typically, when a person meets another, one part of their brain registers the general facial pattern of the person they are meeting. For the person with prosopagnosia, this is a much more involved process. In order to "remember" the other person, he must build the face in his mind. For example, he will have to mentally note that the eyes are asymmetrical and brown or the nose is broad or narrow. Each facial feature must be "entered" into the brain's computer manually. Many don't either know how to do this or just don't bother after a while. This leads to further social isolation.

False Face Recognition

Another problem that can occur with prosopagnosia is false face recognition. The person can think they are remembering correctly, but soon discovers after they have greeted the person that the person is a stranger. This tends to occur more often in younger people as older people with AS have learned to be more cautious in their social interactions.

What You Can Do for Prosopagnosia

The most important thing to do is to determine if you or your child has it. The social deficits associated with AS are difficult enough to contend with, and prosopagnosia just compounds them. But if you realize that you have this, then you can work on strategies to minimize its effect. If your child has it and you work with him to develop coping strategies, his early years will be much happier. Prosopagnosia is either a genetic condition or an incurable neurological one. There is no known medicine or surgical procedure to restore the part of the brain that is malfunctioning. However, there are many coping strategies that can help the person with prospagnosia to mask the condition.

1. Construct the face using a different part of the brain. For example, when meeting someone he wants to remember, one of my patients will process the face manually. He will think, "This person has a slightly large nose with a crook half-inch from the top, the forehead is a little too short for perfect symmetry, the lips are full on the bottom and not on the top," etc. This is extremely time-consuming and tiring, so it wouldn't be used on a regular basis. But it has worked well for many people.

2. If someone looks at you for more than a second and seems to recognize you, then assume you know them and greet them.

3. If you think your child has prosopagnosia, start helping her to see specific nonfacial characteristics of others. For example, Mary smiles a lot and talks loudly, or Tommy often keeps his hands in his pocket and rocks back on his heels. Sally has freckles; Ken wears glasses. You might also alert the teacher who can then use the other student's name and help clue your child as to the identity, especially in the first week or so of the school year.

4. Smile and don't be defensive. One young woman worked eight hours with a coworker chatting about their life stories. Two weeks later, she was assigned to the same store and started to introduce herself only to be rebuffed with an indignant, "We already met." Completely unperturbed, the woman with prosopagnosia laughed and said, "There I go again." She joked about her difficulty with faces and within a few minutes, they started up their earlier conversation.

5. Work out a system with a gregarious friend to always greet the person by name, so you have something to work from. Usually, the person with prospagnosia will start to remember the other person if they have a name and some sort of physical mannerism clue.

6. One great way to develop alternative identifying skills is to sit in a mall and "people watch." People have different gaits and hand mannerisms. They even stand differently. Some hold themselves erect, others slouch, while others shift their weight from one leg to the other. People are often consistent in their basic emotional state. Some are chronically anxious, or always joking, or frequently somber.

7. When you meet someone for the first time, tell them that you have this problem and do not mean offense. There are two variations on this strategy. One AS man in local politics will laughingly be self-deprecating and "give permission" to the other person to call him on this oversight. The other AS person is more clinical and selective about it. When she wants to maintain a business or social connection, she mentions that

she has a neurological condition inherited from her father that makes it difficult for her to remember faces but not conversations with people until she has met the person several times. She encourages the other person when they see her in public to identify themselves first and to attribute her difficulty in recognizing them as a genetic condition rather than unfriendliness or unprofessionalism.

For the person with AS, prosopagnosia is just one piece of the condition's puzzle. What makes it especially challenging is that for the majority of people, other than learn some coping skills, there isn't anything that can be done about it.

Place Blindness: Topographic Agnosia—Always Getting Lost

In some AS people, face blindness (prosopagnosia) may exist alone or be accompanied by place blindness (topographic agnosia). In the adult AS population that I have worked with, about 30 percent seem to have place blindness. There are no national statistics as this condition is often not identified in either the general or in the AS community.

Often confused for being absentminded or lazy, people with topographic agnosia have no innate memory for places. Just as a person with face blindness has a short-term memory for faces, the person with place blindness has a short-term memory for places. This means, that a person living on a street for five years would not be able to recognize the other houses on the street or in the neighborhood if seen out of context. In testing for place blindness, a husband asked his place-blind wife to keep her eyes shut while he drove around their neighborhood. He stopped in front of a house four houses down from theirs and asked her to tell him if she had ever seen it before. She hadn't. Despite their many walks in which they had passed it, she had no memory of it. Topographic agnosia also explains why a person who loved hiking and being out-of-doors would never go by herself and couldn't remember the individual hikes. Unless they included waterfalls or a unique bridge or old growth, all the hikes looked the same to her.

One of the most striking cases of topographic agnosia was of a three-year-old child who was later diagnosed with AS.

Three-year-old Ellen was one of six children. While she seemed to love to be outdoors, unlike her other sisters and brothers, she would not leave the house except with her mom present. Instead, she looked longingly from the back window at her yard. One day, feeling somewhat frustrated, her mom tied a long cord around Ellen's waist and tied the other end loosely to the large tree in the middle of the back yard. Ellen played happily for hours knowing her boundaries. Later, several neighborhood children came by and untied Ellen. Ellen let out a howl and wouldn't stop screaming until her mom rushed out and retied the cord. Decades later, Ellen discovered that not only did she have AS, but she also had a neurological condition that can accompany AS called geographic agnosia or place blindness. She needed that rope, because she was unable to recognize her house versus the next-door neighbor's house. Without that rope, she was lost and had no way to return home. But to others, this appeared as just strange behavior.

Fortunately, for Ellen, her mom trusted her instincts and devised a plan, which while unorthodox, helped her child.

Like face blindness, place blindness is an incredibly frustrating condition. But unlike face blindness, it's harder to hide, especially as an adult. The person with topographic agnosia tends to look forgetful or scatter-brained. The person with topographic agnosia relies on landmarks to get from one location to another. There are no shortcuts, they must go the same way each time, and they must start out at the same location each time. If there is a change in landmarks, such as a change in a billboard, a detour in the road, or hedges cut down, the person can be irretrievably lost. Usually there is no innate sense of direction. Like face blindness, it can vary in intensity. One young man was lost for forty-five minutes two blocks from his new house. Some find maps useless, while others won't leave their home without a map. Each finds a solution. One young man, for whom maps were not helpful, would study a three-dimensional satellite/aerial imagery computer program to get a sense of where he was going. A successful businessman would simply get the managers at the various branches to pick him up from the airport rather than rent a car and try to navigate himself. Another would say out loud the landmarks as she passed them, so that she could process them for her return trip. She relied on her auditory processing because her visual processing was impaired. And whenever possible, she did "dry runs" of the trip, so that there would be fewer instances of getting lost.

Like face blindness, topographical agnosia tends to run in a family. In one family, there were three generations of people with this condition. Only two of them also had AS. While they would joke about the condition, they would always give themselves extra time to get lost for appointments.

What is especially interesting is that while at least half also have face blindness right along with the place blindness, the others seem to have a better than average ability to remember places. One man with severe face blindness was able to successfully navigate the New York subway system in three days. A twenty-one-year-old-man was able to immediately recognize a person he had gone to school with seven years earlier despite the fact that each was about a foot taller, thirty pounds heavier and looked significantly different from their younger selves.

There is little formal research on topographic agnosia. Anecdotal accounts on the Internet abound. Like the preliminary research on prosopagnosia, most of the researchers on topographic agnosia are studying people with brain injuries resulting in this condition. Over the next decade we may see more research in this area. But in the meantime, here are some general recommendations.

1. Always give yourself fifteen to thirty extra minutes for important engagements.
2. Do a dry run, if possible.

3. If you can afford it, get a GPS (Global Positioning System) for your car.
4. Always keep a map in your car.
5. When you are going to a new place, and need to return by the same route, say the names of landmarks out loud. Keep the directions general remembering the name of the street and if possible a landmark such as a gas station, rather than turning right or left as it will be reversed on your return trip. That way, you are using a different part of the brain and have a much greater chance of remembering.

There are no cures or easy solutions for either face blindness or place blindness. Both are incredibly frustrating conditions for both the person with them and those around them. The brain is a remarkable machine that, if trained, can circumvent areas that are not functioning well.

CHAPTER 5

Conventional Asperger Treatment: Then and Now

When Dr. Asperger first recognized this syndrome in 1944, these children with their peculiar behavior seemed exceptional and dramatically different from the norm. What we have discovered in the decades since is that this behavior is not new. When a detailed family history is taken, a similar behavior pattern is seen in previous generations. One patient, Karen, discovered her own Asperger Syndrome (AS) behavior after her ten-year-old son was diagnosed. Looking back in her family tree, she realized that her professor uncle whom she had always regarded as being reclusive and eccentric exhibited many of the AS traits. During his few appearances at family reunions, he would hold people hostage as he talked for hours about specific events in the Civil War. In fact, his siblings seemed to have a system laid down where they would rescue the niece or nephew after twenty minutes. When Karen considered her own parents and siblings, she saw many AS behaviors, though not the full-blown condition.

When we look back historically, we can see AS-like behavior in figures such as Albert Einstein, Isaac Newton, Louis Carroll, Hans Christian Anderson, and Thomas Jefferson. Whether they actually had AS will never be known. But the fact that they had these behaviors clearly demonstrates that the poor social skills and severe aversion to social interactions, the literal-mindedness, and the hyperfocus on a few subjects are traits that didn't start with the handful of subjects first observed by Dr. Asperger. Even more recently, we have many successful people such as Nobel Prize-winning economist Vernon Smith and Satoshi Tajiri, the creator of Pokemon, who have been formally diagnosed with AS.

Despite the discovery of this syndrome, widespread recognition of AS did not occur for many decades. Instead, these children were often misdiagnosed as either schizophrenic or psychotic, and institutionalized. In other cases, the child was gently included in the family, may have been considered handicapped, and gradually adapted to some sort of adult life. Sometimes my patients talk about an uncle or aunt (often unmarried) who never moved out of the home. In other cases, the person developed a profession and devoted themselves exclusively to it. It isn't uncommon to see people with AS traits in academia or in the research department within a corporation.

More recently, there have been giant strides in both the scientific investigation and treatment of AS. For the person with AS, this means there are more options to consider. Most of the research presented in this chapter reflects the study of children rather than adults. This is because similar to ADD (Attention Deficit Disorder), Asperger was first recognized in children and is only recently being diagnosed in adults. This is gradually changing and more studies are looking at adults as well.

TREATMENT OPTIONS

Conventional medicine practitioners such as developmental pediatricians, neurologists, and psychiatrists most often employ psychotropic drugs to decrease the intensity of AS symptoms, especially the anxiety and overreactivity. The field of psychology contains a diversity of practitioners and includes various methods to encourage a moderation of excessive or generally unaccepted behaviors. Natural medicine employs nutrition, homeopathy, herbal medicine, and amino acids, both to balance behavior and thought patterns as well as to support, rather than suppress, the nervous system itself. We are including all three medical systems for two reasons. First, it's a good idea to see what the various options are along with their pros and cons. The better educated people are about their choices, the better choices they make for their own unique situation. I commonly hear from my new patients how relieved they are to know that there is a third choice besides drugs or doing nothing. Second, many people with AS use all three types of treatment simultaneously. There is no one correct way to treat AS as what works well for one person may not for another.

CONVENTIONAL MEDICINE

Conventional medicine uses several classifications of medicines to treat AS: antidepressants, psychostimulants, neuroleptics, and mood-stabilizers. The goal is to target the various aspects of the condition and use the appropriate drug that will best address that particular symptom. As with any medicine, there is a trial period to see if the drug will not only work well for that individual, but also cause the mildest side effects. Often it can take several trials with a couple of drugs to arrive at the best fit.

Anti-depressants

The three categories of antidepressants most frequently used to treat AS are tricyclic antidepressants (TCAs), selective serotonin uptake inhibitors (SSRIs), and serotonin and norepinephrine reuptake inhibitors (SNRIs).

TCAs, such as amitriptyline (Elavil), imipramine (Tofranil), desipramine (Norpramin), and nortriptyline (Aventyl), are used mainly for inattentiveness, hyperactivity, repetitive behavior, preoccupation, sleep dysfunction, and anxiety. Possible side effects are weight gain or loss, nervousness, tremors, abnormal taste, changes in blood glucose levels, nausea, urine retention, diarrhea, constipation, and altered hormones. TCAs may affect testosterone levels. In one study, imipramine and amitriptyline were shown to reduce the concentration of active testosterone.[1] In a population that already tends to have low libidos, the TCAs may be a poor choice for adults. Except for the nervousness and weight fluctuations, most of these side effects are fairly uncommon. A symptom to look out for is changes in blood glucose levels, especially if there is a family history of diabetes or hypoglycemia. Changes in blood glucose levels are frequently accompanied by changes in mood. For example, if the adult or child becomes irritable or shaky three hours after taking the medicine, the drug may be causing a drop in blood sugar levels and he should get into the habit of eating a protein snack about two and a half hours after taking the medicine.

SSRIs, including fluoxetine (Prozac), sertraline (Zoloft), paroxetine (Paxil), fluvoxamine (Luvox), citalopram (Celexa), and escitalopram (Lexapro), address obsessive/compulsive symptoms, depression, and anxiety. For some they work well and significantly decrease these symptoms. The downside to these particular drugs is that they can make the person, overactive, irritable, possibly manic, and sometimes apathetic. In some, they can cause seizures. With children, this is a difficult decision for the parents to make especially in light of the FDA (Food and Drug Administration), November 15, 2004, warning: "The Food and Drug Administration (FDA) today issued a Public Health Advisory announcing a multi-pronged strategy to warn the public about the increased risk of suicidal thoughts and behavior ("suicidality") in children and adolescents being treated with antidepressant medications."[2] This occurs especially in the first few months of treatment.

Like, TCAs, SSRIs can affect sexual hormones. Research report, fluoxetine (Prozac) decreased testosterone levels resulting in low libido and apathy.[3] In another study, "Citalopram (Celexa) ... increased significantly the serum testosterone concentration...."[4]

Occasionally, I may have a new patient come in looking extremely dull and apathetic. The parents tell me of a vibrant child who just couldn't seem to conform to the school's behavioral rules. The SSRIs helped the child to moderate her behavior in the school environment, but this also resulted in a dull child. While some children are very happy with the control these medications give them, other children will often tell me the drug makes them feel different from themselves.

Psychostimulants

Psychostimulants are used to improve attention and decrease impulsivity. They are most often employed for the AD(H)D component of AS. Some common psychostimulants are amphetamine (Adderall), pemoline (Cylert), and methylphenidate (Ritalin and Concerta). They can adversely affect the appetite and sleep, and in some cases, increase irritability and depression as well as obsessive and compulsive behaviors such as picking and tics. For many decades, scientists were concerned about its long-term effects. An article published in 1983 in the *Archives of General Psychiatry* by Mattes and Gittelman noted a significant decrease in height percentile after two to four years of using methylphenidate.[5] There was a follow-up article in the same publication in 1988 with similar results based on a second group of children.[6] A 2004 study in the *Journal of Clinical Psychopharmacology* by Wilens, Biederman, and Lerner from Harvard Medical School, examined the effects of long-term use of once-daily osmotic-release methylphenidate (Concerta) on children from six to thirteen years old.[7] They concluded that over a twelve-month period, there were "statistically significant changes in blood pressure and heart rate" in these children. This can be a concern as high blood pressure often occurs anyway in the AS population from years of sustaining severe anxiety levels. Prolonged use of Ritalin or Concerta may hasten or worsen development of high blood pressure.

Amphetamines in general, can cause tics, eye rolling, hand and finger movement, or erratic behavior. One young man threw a chair and swept the contents of a table onto the floor at the end of a tutoring session after starting on Adderal. Upset, remorseful, and terrified about the loss of control, he discontinued the Adderall. The trade-off of improved attention wasn't worth the emotional dysfunction. Pemoline (Cylert), an older drug used for Attention Deficit Hyperactivity Disorder (ADHD)can cause life-threatening liver failure.

Selective Norepinephrine Reuptake Inhibitor

Possibly recognizing the problems with prolonged use of psychostimulants, the pharmaceutical industry developed atomoxetine (Strattera), which was approved by the FDA for children and adults in 2002. Strattera was proclaimed the first nonstimulant drug designed to treat AD(H)D. The WHO (World Health Organization) has a different opinion. It classifies atomoxetine (Strattera) as a central acting sympathomimetic or psychostimulant, and in the same category as methylphenidate (Ritalin).[8] Strattera works by increasing norepinephrine, an adrenal hormone that directly affects attention, concentration, cognition, mood, emotions, and blood pressure. It is involved with maintaining the fight or flight response. Its most common side effects are upset stomach, decreased appetite, nausea or vomiting, constipation, dizziness, tiredness, mood swings, mania, problems in sleeping, sexual side effects, problems urinating, menstrual cramps, and suicidal thinking. FDA-approved in 2002, Strattera received its first FDA warning for the potential side effect of severe liver disease in December 2004.[9] Though this will be discussed in greater detail in the next chapter, often the liver function is suboptimal in conditions such as AS on the autism spectrum. Putting any additional strain on the liver would be something to consider carefully. In September 2005, the United States Food and Drug Administration directed Eli Lilly, the manufacturer of atomoxetine (Strattera), to add a boxed warning and additional warning statements concerning an increased risk of suicidal thinking in children and adolescents when using this drug.[10] This suicidal thinking occurred in the first few months of starting Strattera and happened in less than 1 percent of the cases reviewed.

In the journal, *Pediatrics* dated September 3, 2004, psychiatrists, Drs. Henderson and Hartman, claimed that there was frequent mood destabilization in patients taking Strattera.[11] Out of 153 youths in their practice on Strattera, one-third developed extreme irritability, aggression, or mania. Eighty percent of the youths who experienced mood destabilization had histories of mood symptoms. However, 11 percent had no history of mood symptoms.

There is also an interesting debate among researchers as to whether Strattera is appropriate for those with anxiety. A 2005 University of Nebraska study published in the *Journal of the American Academy of Child and Adolescent Psychiatry* demonstrated its efficacy in treating children with both ADHD and anxiety.[12] A similar study published in the *Journal of Child and Adolescent Psychopharmacology* reported strong positive results in children with Pervasive Developmental Disorder (PDD), another autism spectrum condition similar to AS. The article concludes, "However, children with PDD may have a higher vulnerability for some of the known side-effects of atomoxetine." On the opposing side of the debate are psychiatrists like Grace E. Jackson, author of *Rethinking Psychiatric Drugs*. She suggests people consider whether the physiological mechanism of this medication, to maintain the fight or flight response, and its long-term effects of heart disease, are worth the short-term gains.[13] There is little dispute that Strattera may be beneficial for attention and focus, but it may not be the best medication for people with a naturally heightened fight or flight response such as those with AS.

Another concern with Strattera is its propensity to trigger mania. If you think of mania as racing thoughts, decreased need for sleep, and impulsive, reckless behavior, you can readily see how this would exacerbate AS children's tendency to have violent outbursts. A 2006 study involving children with ADHD by the manufacturer Eli Lilly excluded all those with histories of bipolar disease and seizures.[14] This omission seems an acknowledgment of this potential to cause mania. In order to adjust for this, many psychiatrists are concurrently using mood stabilizers with any person with a history of mania.

While Strattera can be very beneficial for some people, the most common complaint I hear in my office is loss of imagination. Children using Strattera, more so than the adults, often have a dull look to their faces.

Neuroleptics

Neuroleptics, also known as antipsychotics and routinely used in the treatment of schizophrenia, affect dopamine or dopamine and serotonin receptors and can significantly improve a multitude of AS symptoms including social anxiety, overreactivity, attentiveness, stabilize the mood, and decrease aggression. Neuroleptics such as haloperidol (Haldol), chlorpromazine (Thorazine), and especially, risperidone (Risperdal), and aripiprazole (Abilify), have become the first choice medicines in treating AS. Their side effects include, sedation, weight gain, irritability, seizures, tardive dyskinesia (involuntary abnormal movements), and insulin resistance. In rare instances, it can make the body become still and hot with a life-threatening condition called neuroleptic malignant syndrome. According to Dr. Benzer of Harvard Medical School and Massachusetts General Hospital, neuroleptic malignant syndrome can occur "in rates ranging from 0.02–12.2 percent of patients treated with a neuroleptic medication".[15] Many of these side effects can be minimized if the medication is introduced very slowly and decreased with the first sign of an adverse effect. Also, when a person has been using neuroleptics for long periods, it's best to very gradually taper off the medication in order to avoid developing tardive dyskinesia. Tardive dyskinesia includes grimacing, tongue protrusion, lip smacking, puckering and pursing, and rapid eye blinking, and often persists after the neuroleptic drugs have been discontinued. Again, each person must weigh the benefits versus the side effects.

Mood-stabilizers

Mood-stabilizers or what was formerly called antiseizure medicines including valproate (Depakote), carbamazepine (Tegretol), and lithium are also routinely used in treating AS behavior. They treat aggression and seizures and generally balance the overall mood of the person. In some people, these can cause a multitude of side effects including, confusion, fatigue, blood abnormalities, abdominal pain, liver disorders, joint pain, and heart irregularities. While there is very little research on the use of mood stabilizers with autism spectrum conditions, there is reason to be cautious. In one article, the authors "report a case of new-onset epileptic seizures induced by carbamazepine in an individual with autism spectrum disorders (ASD)." They urge clinicians to consider " . . . the possibility that epileptic seizures may possibly be either precipitated or exacerbated by carbamazepine especially in individuals with ASD."[16]

Alpha-2 Adrenergic Agonists (Blood Pressure Drugs)

A new direction for AS treatment comes in the form of using medications commonly prescribed for high blood pressure such as guanfacine (Tenex). It decreases the "fight or flight" sympathetic nervous system that is so prominent in the AS population. Possible side effects are confusion, depression, drowsiness, decreased libido, skin conditions, constipation, and mania. A 1999 article by Horrigan and Barnhill in the *Journal of Affective Disorders* discussed the secondary mania that occurred in study participants with either a personal or a family history of bipolar disorder.[17] Because these two conditions can exist together in both children and adults, guanfacine should be avoided in these situations.

USING MULTIPLE MEDICATIONS AND DETERMINING POSSIBLE SIDE EFFECTS

It's a common practice to have a person on multiple drugs to treat the AS behavior. For example, Tenex, a blood pressure medication used to decrease the fight or flight anxiety may be used in conjunction with the antipsychotic olanzapine (Zyprexa), and the antidepressant, citalopram (Celexa). Because of this, it's important to be aware of their probable interactions. One way to determine the interactions is to compare the inserts of the medications or go to the library and compare the adverse reactions in either the PDR (physician's desk reference) or the nurses' counterpart to this book. If there is the same adverse effect in more than one medicine, the chance of developing that side effect increases. Many times the adverse effect will develop and the prescribing physician will simply add another drug to address the side effect. Each drug adds a new potential for additional side effects. For example, SSRIs and neuroleptics can cause seizures. If that happens, an antiseizure medication may be added to the treatment plan and an even greater potential for additional side effects occurs.

Most people are more susceptible to the medical conditions that occur in their own families. For example, let's say the parents or grandparents of the AS person using the medications have heart disease but no arthritis. The AS medications list heart-related conditions and joint pain as potential adverse effects. The more likely side effect to occur in the person is the heart-related condition and not the joint pain.

Additionally, it's important to consider the long-term effect of these medications on the liver and the heart. In most cases, there haven't been long-term studies of the effects of taking these medications for years. Often the medications being used haven't been studied specifically for the AS population. While in some cases they are extremely beneficial, there are many safer and as effective options in natural medicine.

OVERALL EFFECT OF MEDICATIONS ON CHILDREN

Conventional drugs generally don't make children behave in a normal fashion; they simply moderate the extreme behavior. And while this might be necessary for a short duration, it's important to give your children the tools to manage themselves better at the same time. Consider if you are giving your child medication because of pressure from teachers and well-meaning family members. When deciding whether or not to medicate your child, it's important to factor in the probable weight gain, the subsequent peer-teasing from the weight gain, and the increased risk of diabetes, and determine if there are either different medications without these side effects to address the condition, or if other forms of treatment may be more appropriate. Perhaps the most important medical consideration is that we know so little about the effects of these medications on AS.

COMING OFF CONVENTIONAL MEDICATIONS

Once conventional medication is stopped expect an increase in anger, which had been previously masked by the medication. This can be seen in adults, but it is more often seen in children. If you decide to stop your medication, please consult your prescribing doctor and do it very slowly. The most successful way to wean off antidepressants is to decrease it slowly over three months so that there are little to no side effects. The slower the process, the less risk of relapse. Here are some symptoms that may occur when withdrawing from TCAs and SSRI/SNRIs antidepressants:

1. TCAs: Anxiety, anorexia, nausea, vomiting, diarrhea, sweating, headache, chills, lethargy, insomnia, vivid dreams, mania, hypomania, panic attacks, delirium, and cardiac arrythmias.[18]
2. SSRI/SNRIs: Flu-like symptoms, dizziness, headache, electric shocks, insomnia, vertigo, memory problems, tremor, mania, suicidality, night-mares, irritability, impulsivity, crying spells, and anxiety.[19]

While conventional medicine plays a important role in the treatment of AS, there are many mental health disciplines and other nonmedical treat-ment options in addressing the person with AS. Practitioners of these disci-plines may include clinical psychologists, social workers, occupational therapists, physical therapists, speech pathologists, and audiologists. Several of these dis-ciplines overlap, but the following is a brief description of the work various therapists do.

CLINICAL PSYCHOLOGISTS

Clinical Psychologists are licensed mental health professional (Ph.D. or Psy.D.) who evaluate, diagnosis, and treat mental health conditions. Psychologists diag-nose conditions using cognitive, academic, and personality testing. Each clinical psychologist generally specializes in treating one or two areas of mental health such as depression, posttraumatic stress disorder, or obsessive-compulsive disor-der, and often target one age group. They may work individually with the person or in a family or group setting. In addition, clinical psychologists ascribe to various methods of psychological therapies including behavioral analysis, cognitive ther-apy, behavioral cognitive therapy, and problem solving. The following is a brief overview of the major forms of psychological therapy that are useful for people with AS.

Behavioral Analysis

In Behavioral Analysis, the therapist works with the client to set specific objectives focused on the unlearning of negative behavior and replacing them with productive behavior. This is a fairly structured format and includes regular homework assignments to incorporate what is learned in the sessions. It is often applied to treat anxiety and obsessive-compulsive tendencies.

Problem-Solving

This therapy has a narrower focus. It targets specific stresses that contribute to depression and anxiety, ranks them in importance, and then works on them one at a time. Emphasizing self-reliance, this method is designed to both address the current stresses in the patient's life as well as give the patient a tool to handle future stresses.

Cognitive Therapy

Based on the theory that how you think affects how you feel, cognitive therapy seeks to alter thought patterns. For example, the patient learns to challenge anxiety-producing thoughts in ten to fifteen fifty-minute weekly sessions plus homework assignments. The goal is to think more realistically, which results in feeling better.

Cognitive Behavioral Therapy (CBT)

As the name suggests, this therapy is directed toward setting objective realistic goals for changes in both the thought and behavioral patterns of the client. Within CBT are multiple techniques such as challenging irrational beliefs, assertiveness, and social skills training.

SOCIAL WORKERS

Social workers help patients with emotional and physical needs in the day-to-day aspects of their patients' lives. They may offer suggestions for crisis in the family, school, or workplace. They are often a resource to direct people with AS to the appropriate community services. There are several categories of social workers. For example, a clinical social worker (MSW) has a master's degree in certain psychiatric techniques and specializes in mental health. A licensed clinical social worker has the same academic education as the MSW but has successfully completed two years of supervised clinical experience and has received a license from the state board acknowledging this additional education.

Social workers are very effective in situations when there are multiple dynamics going on. For example, when a teenager has diagnosed AS, the mom has OCD (obsessive compulsive disorder), and the dad has undiagnosed AS. These situations can be highly inflammatory. The social worker can help mediate a less stressful situation.

OCCUPATIONAL THERAPISTS (OT)

An occupational therapist is someone who helps an adult or child to do his job, whether that job is play, study, or work.

Children

In the school setting, the occupational therapist helps children with basic sensory, motor, neuromuscular, and/or visual skills. This is especially important in AS in which fine or gross motor skill deficits are common. For example, an occupational therapist may teach the AS child fine motor skills such as how to hold a pen or pencil correctly. They may work on gross motor coordination to help the often clumsy AS child have an easier time in PE (physical education) classes by using swings and trampolines to help with coordination. They can help with ocular skills in children who lose their place while reading or miss words. One of the most important areas with which occupational therapists are involved is Sensory Processing. In virtually every aspect of our lives, our senses of hearing, sight, smell, taste, and touch send messages to our brain to make us aware of what is going on in each situation. For example, if a burner is hot, our brains send out a signal and we don't touch it. Because AS is a neurological condition, in some people with AS, the complex neurological processes that control the senses aren't functioning well, resulting in impaired Sensory Processing. Their brains are relaying an inaccurate assessment of the situation. For example, the person's sensory receptors may be understimulated and not register pain. In other cases, it may be overstimulated in which common foods, textures, and smells are offensive or even painful to the person. In other cases, some AS children and adults tend to startle easily. The occupational therapist can work on sensory issues by gradually desensitizing a child to common textures to which the child has an aversion. The occupational therapist will encourage the parent to incorporate the same exercises done in school at home to both reinforce the lesson and to help the child improve more quickly.

Adults

The occupational therapist's focus when working with adults is directed toward sensory processing and proprioception or the innate awareness of the different parts of one's body. Just as its name indicates, sensory processing focuses on the five senses of sight, smell, taste, touch, and sound. Proprioception is similar to these senses but it relates to the body's unconscious ability to respond to incoming information. For example, poor proprioception would cause a person to grip a pencil too tightly or touch something too hot. Here's an example of how an occupational therapist may help someone with AS.

There was an AS computer programmer who would wear a hat, sunglasses, and earplugs at work to decrease distraction. This coping mechanism was hindering her chances of promotion despite excellent work. After the occupational therapist accessed the situation, she determined that the programmer had sensory and proprioception difficulties. The OT suggested a couple of exercises that involved heavy work input, which included wall pushups and carrying heavy items for a few minutes each morning prior to going to work. These exercises grounded the programmer, helping her to have better focus. In addition, the programmer gradually desensitized herself in the privacy of her own home by sitting under the fluorescent lights in the kitchen and reading while the TV was on. At first she could only tolerate this for five minutes, but gradually, she learned to start tuning things out and was able to read. She was also given a stress ball to help stay focused.

The OT develops a plan individual for each person that is designed to help balance whatever visual, motor, sensory, or postural concern the person may have.

PHYSICAL THERAPISTS

This form of therapy can be as formal or informal as the parents want. Physical therapists may provide various forms of exercise and physical activities to help with coordination and body awareness. They may use water, aerobic, or breathing exercises. These exercises often integrate body and mind to help improve concentration, memory, reading, writing, organizing, listening, as well as physical coordination. There is a certain amount of overlap between occupational therapists and physical therapists when treating people with AS. Occupational therapists have a more comprehensive approach and help to minimize neurological dysfunctions in the school, home, and workplace whereas physical therapists more often address gross motor coordination.

SPEECH PATHOLOGISTS

Trained to evaluate, diagnose, and treat adults and children with swallowing and speech problems, speech pathologists may be helpful with AS children not because they don't speak well, but because they often don't speak functionally. Their speech pragmatics is deficient. Speech pragmatics involves understanding how to appropriately speak in various circumstances. For example, how to speak to a child versus an adult, or knowing how to take turns in conversing with others. The AS child may speak in a pedantic, stiff manner that doesn't invite a normal give-and-take with other children. The speech pathologist can help teach the AS child or adult how to verbally interact with others in a better way.

AUDIOLOGISTS

Typically, audiologists evaluate hearing loss. Some children and adults with AS have central auditory processing dysfunction or a difficulty in hearing and interpreting words accurately. Many teachers and parents confuse this with ADD. In ADD, the person has trouble staying focused because his attention wanders. In central auditory processing dysfunction, the person actually has trouble isolating voices and mishears words. They will have trouble following multiple-step directions and will appear confused in conversations. Even when words are spoken clearly and slowly, the person might need additional time to process the sentence as he can only hear words or consonants in a jumbled fashion. Audiologists, therefore, play a more integral role in the AS community. Using an experimental technique called Auditory Integration Training, audiologists strive to decrease the painful sensitivity to sound that exists in many AS children and in some AS adults. It also helps the child or adult filter out extraneous sounds so that they can improve their listening skills.

In addition to the more traditional therapies discussed above, there are a host of different adjunct therapies, which have other benefits. These are covered in Chapter 11.

CHAPTER 6

Physical Symptoms Associated with Asperger Syndrome

Since the most debilitating symptoms of Asperger Syndrome (AS) are anxiety, social awkwardness, and overreactivity, most people look for solutions at a mental health professional's office. The mental health professional will diagnose the condition and explain that AS is a condition requiring treatment to balance an overactive nervous system. It seems logical to treat a neurological condition with medications targeting the nervous system. Our western conventional medicine supports this belief. Most physicians are specialists who treat one part of the person. For example, a neurologist would see a person for a condition affecting the nervous system, while a gastroenterologist would see the same person for any digestive condition. Generally there isn't any communication between the different physicians, and while that might work for some conditions, in AS, it can limit the ability of the person to dramatically improve.

Despite its classification as a neurological condition, AS affects multiple systems in the body. It is common to see a physical pattern emerge right alongside the more well known symptoms of anxiety, social dysfunction, and overreactivity. High blood pressure, hypoglycemia, constipation, diarrhea, headaches, fungal skin and intestinal conditions, food sensitivities or allergies especially to wheat and sugar, sleep irregularities as well as more serious digestive disorders, are a common part of the AS picture. The adult will often have two to four concurrent physical concerns that they either have adapted to or simply don't associate with AS. In fact, I have patients who tell me their digestion is fine and then admit to taking occasional antacids, eating prunes or fiber pills, not having a bowel movement daily, or having bad-smelling bowel movements. These are all indications that the digestive tract isn't working well. When the doctor treats the whole person, the AS symptoms stabilize much faster. Here's a short true-false quiz that gives an indication of the health of your digestion.

1. I have or have had periods of diarrhea or not having a daily bowel movement.
2. I have some gas or tend to bloat after eating.
3. Often my stomach doesn't feel right after I eat.
4. As a child, I have or had routine stomachaches.
5. I take over-the-counter or prescription antacids.
6. I can't go for very long without eating or my anxiety gets worse or I get shaky and feel irritable.
7. I have or have had medical conditions related to my digestive tract such as Irritable Bowel Syndrome, Crohn's Disease, or colitis.
8. I have high blood pressure.
9. I tend to eat sweet foods or drinks such as pop or soda or fruit juice daily.
10. I have or have had bouts of athlete's foot or toenail discoloration.
11. I have had several bouts of yeast infections or jock itch.
12. I have or have had bouts of persistent minor skin conditions that don't seem to respond to antibacterial ointment.
13. I get headaches and suspect that they may be related to something I'm eating.

If you have AS, then it is likely that you will answer "true" to six or more of these questions. Most people with AS don't realize that these may all be part of the AS picture and as the body, specifically the digestion improves, the AS symptoms decrease. In fact, in young children with AS, I find that the parents are bringing them in for digestive concerns sometimes for years before the formal diagnosis.

TREATING THE HEAD BY HEALING THE GUT

The digestive tract plays a crucial role in the AS condition. If you think of the digestive tract as a long tube starting with your mouth and ending with your anus, you can see that there are plenty of areas where problems can occur. For example, we are seeing heartburn and stomachaches from poor digestion in AS children as young as three-years-old. We know the digestive tract's health affects not only how comfortable you feel after a meal, but your immune function and very likely AS psychological symptoms. Most of the research in this chapter is based on autism studies and extrapolated to AS since it is a closely related condition. Clinicians treating Asperger Syndrome are finding that their young patients routinely have constipation or diarrhea, gassiness and bloating, reflux, and sensitivities to one or more foods, most frequently dairy, sugar, or wheat. And in adults they may see these same symptoms plus irritable bowel disorder and various inflammatory conditions such as Crohn's and Inflammatory Bowel disease. In a 2002 study for the National Institute of Health, Kevin Becker et al. identified identical genetic markers linked to both autism and celiac disease and autism and Crohn's Disease.[1] This is one possible explanation why intestinal conditions are so routinely seen in Asperger patients. Research by scientists

Martha Welch et al. is looking at the brain effects of inflammatory bowel disease. Their work advances the idea that an inflammatory bowel condition can lead to secondary neural changes.[2] This supports the idea that our intestinal health affects our behavior health. Horvath and Perman from the University of Baltimore School of Medicine in a 2002 article report on "Three surveys conducted in the United States described high prevalence of gastrointestinal symptoms in children with autistic disorder."[3] They describe the abnormalities in the intestinal lining and the liver's ability to break down toxic substances so they can pass out of the body, in the autistic population. One of the abnormalities these researchers are alluding to is "leaky gut." An important concept in understanding how the intestinal health affects the overall health, the "leaky gut" theory proposes that people with poor digestion have intestinal permeability or gaps in the gut cell lining. These gaps allow proteins, bacteria, and toxins to pass into the blood stream instead of remaining in the digestive tract and being excreted in the stool. Once these substances enter the blood stream, they can cause a host of symptoms ranging from headaches, itchy eyes, runny nose, joint pain, to skin eruptions, as well as various inflammatory intestinal problems. What many doctors who treat AS are finding is that when they heal the intestinal problems, not only does the physical health benefit, but the ability to focus and the overall emotional state also improve.

> Rachel was a exuberant 10 year-old girl who came to my office with severe constipation. Her favorite food was pasta and she would eat a large plate of it every night, often without eating any of the rest of the dinner. She had already been to the emergency room 2 times with impaction when her bowels had simply shut down. Despite her extreme outgoing nature, Rachel was plagued by anxiety, often over-reacted, had virtually no friends, and had been diagnosed as ADHD. As I treated her bowels, I suggested that she be evaluated for Asperger Syndrome. And though the eventual AS diagnosis was a big surprise to her mother, I explained how digestive problems and Asperger Syndrome seem to go hand-in-hand. Happily, as her bowels healed, her ADHD and anxiety symptoms decreased as well

Some of the most compelling research to support the integral relationship between AS, part of the autism spectrum, and the health of the intestines came from a controversial examination of the effects of vaccinations on the intestinal health of the autistic community. When the world-respected British medical journal, *The Lancet*, first published Andrew Wakefield's findings connecting gastrointestinal conditions with autism via vaccinations, it offered a scientific explanation for how this digestive tract damage related to the extreme behaviors in children and adults.[4] Since then, Wakefield's research has been supported by many other scientists.[5, 6] Even more importantly to the person with AS, doctors see a dramatic improvement in the behaviors of both their children and adult patients by focusing on the health of the intestines in their clinics.

Sometimes, in AS adults, the emphasis is so strongly on medication for the anxiety and subsequent depression, that the digestive problems seem secondary. They may have feet of intestines cut out, live on antacids or laxatives, and often not see a connection with their anxiety, ability to focus, and depression. If you answered yes to several of the questions above, then consider working on your digestion. Here are some common digestive problems in the AS community and some general recommendations to treat them.

LOW STOMACH ACID

The stomach naturally secretes hydrochloric acid to break down food and kill off harmful substances like bacteria that might come in with the food. If you think of the stomach as a blender, it might give you a better idea of how it works. With hydrochloric acid acting like the blades, the food is churned until it is broken down enough to enter the small intestine. If your stomach doesn't produce enough hydrochloric acid, the food doesn't break down adequately. The food then enters the small intestines in such large pieces that it is difficult for the small intestines to absorb nutrients. For example, even if you eat a really healthy meal but don't have enough hydrochloric acid, then you won't absorb some of the nutrients in the food. These nutrients such as the B-vitamins and minerals such as magnesium, calcium, and potassium are essential for a healthy nervous system. Just as bad, if you have a leaky gut or intestinal permeability, when the food does reach the intestines in a larger form, then it will allow toxins, harmful proteins, and bacteria to get into the blood stream. Some readers will be thinking, "I have the opposite problem, too much hydrochloric acid." Maybe not. Acid reflux is often a combination of insufficient hydrochloric acid taking too long to break down food coupled with a faulty backflow valve from your esophagus. As numerous holistic doctors, including Dr. Jonathan Wright, have discovered in clinical practice, many people with acid reflux do extremely well with a tablespoon of apple cider vinegar or lemon water before meals. Symptoms of low hydrochloric acid include bloating, burping, offensive stools, flatulence, and tiredness after meals. These symptoms are not exclusively from low stomach acid but may be an indication of it.

How to Test for Low Stomach Acid

If you have several of the symptoms for low stomach acid, there are various ways your doctor can test for hypochlorhydria or low stomach acid. One of them involves swallowing and then pulling back out a pH-sensitive capsule attached to a string. However, a simple home test is to drink a tablespoon of fresh lemon juice or apple cider vinegar on an empty stomach. If you have sufficient hydrochloric acid (HCl), you will feel mildly nauseous within a few minutes. This nausea can easily be relieved by water and a cracker. The lemon triggered the stomach acid secretion but when food didn't follow the lemon, the secreted hydrochloric acid had nothing to break down, resulting in nausea. If you don't feel nauseous or even queasy, then you probably don't produce enough hydrochloric acid. The same test can be done when you have heartburn. If it is quickly relieved, then you have too little HCl.

Treatment for Low Stomach Acid—(Do Only One of These Suggestions at a Time)

1. One to two tablespoons lemon juice or one tablespoon of apple cider vinegar before meals.
2. 750 mg–2000 mg of betaine hydrochloric acid pills with each meal for adults. I tend to give herbs or lemon juice to children.
3. Bitter herbs such as goldenseal and gentian. These two herbs are more effective in liquid form. They don't work if given in pill form as they won't produce a sour taste, which triggers receptors in the mouth leading to the secretion of gastrin, a hormone in the stomach that stimulates the secretion of HCl. Both of these herbs are very bitter, so they need to be taken in quarter to one teaspoon doses or mixed with ginger or cinnamon.

Bloating, Flatulence, and General Digestive Discomfort

Sometimes, insufficient hydrochloric acid is only part of the problem. The person will complain of bloating, too much gas, and a general uncomfortable feeling after eating. All of these reflect insufficient enzymes. In children, it can be too few enzymes, despite sufficient hydrochloric acid. After the stomach acid breaks down the food, it moves into the small intestine, where the valuable nutrients are taken out. It's at this stage that enzymes come into play. There are many different kinds of enzymes and multiple subclassifications of each enzyme. Most people grab a bottle off a shelf based on the label without understanding what the product will actually do. They bring it home and find it works sometimes or sometimes not at all. Enzymes can become complicated and confusing quickly. The key is to understand what digestive or metabolic process the various enzymes target and then to find a formulation that is appropriate for your situation. Amylase, invertase (sucrase), glucoamylase, maltase, and phytase all break down carbohydrates. Lactase breaks down milk sugars and is needed for dairy allergies or intolerances. Protease, papain, and bromelain break down protein. However, bromelain is much less effective than protease and it is used more for inflammation and pain when taken on an empty stomach. There are many types of protease enzymes, so when looking for an enzyme product, see if it contains a protease blend. Lipase breaks down fat and helps the body to use it more effectively. The best formulations for those with AS are the ones in which there are several forms of protease enzymes, as wheat and gluten intolerances, common in this population, are most effectively treated by these types of enzymes.

But getting the correct enzymes is just the first part of the process. Enzymes can require different pH, acid-base balance, in the intestines. Protease, lipase, and amylase or plant-based enzymes can break down fat, protein, and carbohydrates in a broader pH range than other type enzymes. This is important in that some enzyme companies promote enzymes such as chymotrypsin, or pepsin, which need certain pHs in order to be effective and may be killed off in more acidic parts of the body such as the stomach.

If you see other enzymes on the bottle, it's good to know their purposes. For example, the enzyme catalase helps decompose excess hydrogen peroxide, which can damage cells, or nattokinase is more specific for heart health, including decreasing triglycerides and cholesterol and might be completely unnecessary for a young child, but helpful for an adult. There is a huge difference in quality and formulations. There are different measuring units for enzymes, so it's often difficult to compare the amount of one brand to another. It's best to purchase only good quality enzymes from reputable companies that make targeted enzyme formulations for different digestive problems. Again, please don't assume that large corporations make better products. I don't find that to be true very often. Your natural health practitioner will know the companies that sell superior quality enzymes and I have listed a couple in the Appendix that are available in your local health food store. I'm going into this much detail so that you use caution when choosing an enzyme and get the one that is the most effective for you.

Enzymes are complicated. Karen DeFelice writes one of the clearest explanations of enzymes and their effect on the body as pertaining to AS in her book, *Enzymes for Autism and Other Neurological Conditions*. She discusses how to use enzymes and what to expect while you are determining which enzymes are needed.

Intestinal Candidiasis

Approximately 75 percent of all the AS children I treat and 50 percent of the adults have an overgrowth of intestinal fungi, which most people refer to as candida. *Candida albicans* is the most common fungi that can be overgrown, but it is not the only one. *Candida tropicalis, Candida parapsilosis, Candida guilliermondi*, and *Torulopsis glabrata* are others that can cause similar disruption to healthy digestion. In children, there may be a history of multiple rounds of antibiotics, a persistent diaper rash, recurrent thrush, or miscellaneous skin rashes. Silly behavior and sugar cravings are also signs of this condition. One AS teenage boy would giggle in his physics class. This was not only embarrassing but also puzzling to him. He also had a persistent skin rash that defied conventional treatment. Both the rash and the giggling stopped after he was successfully treated for candida.

In adults with candida, I look for multiple rounds of antibiotics, cortisone use, recurrent athletes' foot, jock itch or vaginal candida, chronic sinusitis, birth control pills, and a strong sweet tooth. Not only do these physical conditions clear up with treatment, but the person also seems more emotionally stable.

The treatment for intestinal candida is three-pronged: diet, probiotics, and antifungals. The candida diet cuts off the supply of food that feeds the candida and the antifungals kill the excess fungi in the intestines. The probiotics increase the intestine's supply of beneficial bacteria, which keep the fungal overgrowth in check. All three must be done concurrently and for at least two months to correct the condition.

The candida diet consists of eliminating sugar in any form, vinegars, and yeast-containing foods. Sugar is more than just white table sugar, honey, maple syrup, corn syrup, and barley malt. It also includes alcohol, juices, dried fruit, and catsup. A single pear or apple a day doesn't seem to affect the candida. Sugar is added to virtually every processed food, so read labels. Even better, cook from scratch so you know what you are eating. And yes, for this treatment, alcohol in any form is on the sugar list and should be avoided during the candida treatment. Yeast includes those found in breads and other baked goods as well as nutritional yeast included as a flavoring in many processed foods.

The second part of this antifungal treatment is probiotics. Like most supplements, probiotics vary significantly in quality. The two things to look for are variety and amounts of friendly bacteria. The most common probiotic strain is *acidophilus bifidus*. However, a good probiotic is refrigerated and will have at least six to twelve different strains in it. Other strains include *lactobacillus rhamnosus*, *acidophilus*, *casei*, *plantarum*, *salivarius*, and *bifidobacterium bifidum*, *longum*, *infantis*, and *brevis*. A single dose should contain ten to twenty-five billion units depending on whether treating a child or an adult. Many people ask about the probiotics that aren't refrigerated. I recommend them only for travel, as they are less consistent in their amounts. Probiotics decompose at room temperature. Though there is debate about when to take probiotics, they seem to be most effective when taken on an empty stomach so they can pass quickly into the small intestines.

The final prongs to the intestinal candida treatment are antifungal herbs or other supplements. For the average intestinal fungal overgrowth, conventional medical treatments such as nystatin or fluconazole aren't really necessary and are appropriate for only the most persistent cases. These conventional drugs are excellent in killing off the candida but don't repopulate with friendly bacteria or address the cause of the problem. Also, the possible adverse effects of these drugs, nausea, diarrhea, headache, vomiting, rash, hives, fatigue, and its negative effect on the liver outweigh the benefit in all but the most persistent cases. And, the drugs become less and less effective the more times they are repeated.

Three common antifungal herbs that have been shown both in laboratory testing and clinical use to be effective are *Tabebuia spp.* (Pau d'arco), *Usnea spp.* (Old Man's Beard), and *Spilanthes acmella* (Paracress). Each herb targets some rather than all fungi, so it's best if used in combination. For example, *Tabebuia* works well against *candida albicans*,[7] *Spilanthes* targets various Aspergillus forms of fungi,[8] while *Usnea* is traditionally used to treat candida species and seems to be a more broad-spectrum antifungal. This doesn't mean that these herbs, in combination, won't help with other fungi, it just means that these are the ones that scientists have tested for. Other natural substances well known for their antifungal properties, caprylic acid, grapefruit seed extract, garlic, ginger, and oregano oil all have well-researched antifungal qualities and are frequently found in antifungal supplements. For a more effective antifungal treatment, use a combination of these natural substances.

Safety of Herbs

Occasionally, someone will question the safety of natural medicine, specifically herbs. They wonder if herbs don't have the same amount of side effects that seem to plague conventional drugs, but just haven't been researched enough. Herbs have been used and studied for thousands of years. Over this time, the herbs with serious side effects have been identified. In modern herbal medicine, we call these herbs "low dose botanicals" and use them infrequently and with caution. Many old and modern herbal texts give specific ranges for safe dosages of herbs and discuss the possible long-term effects. A physician trained in herbal medicine knows how long and in what quantities to use a herb. The caution with herbs is twofold. First, when they are used without guidance, and second with poor manufacturing practices. Herbs do not have the same action as conventional drugs. Consider the white willow bark. It's a natural pain reliever containing acetylsalicylic acid, the chemical constituent of aspirin. In addition to the acetylsalicylic acid, white willow bark also contains antiinflammatory bioflavonoids components that protect the intestinal lining. The pharmaceutical industry developed the one constituent of the plant into the drug aspirin, but didn't include the other protective constituents. This resulted in the ulcer-producing effect of aspirin. White willow bark doesn't cause ulcers.

Sometimes, someone will come in with chronic yeast infections whether athletes' foot or vaginal, chronic, sinusitis, and craves sugar. This is a more serious fungi infiltration. For this group, I also recommend a blend of protease and cellulase enzymes, which break down the cell walls of the fungi. You can find more information on this in the Appendix.

When starting a candida treatment, it's best to proceed slowly. Eliminate all obvious sugars over a period of a week and then pull out the less obvious. Start the probiotics and herbs with one dose daily and increase to two doses depending on how you feel. If you start the treatment abruptly, you or your child will experience "die-off" or the Herxheimer reaction. Die-off can consist of brain fog, nausea, a sense of being intoxicated, and headache. This can be completely avoided if the process is done gradually over a period of one week. Die-off is a reaction to the candida decomposing in the intestines and getting into the blood stream. The more gradual the process, the more the body, specifically the liver, can handle this process without discomfort.

Another thing to watch for is sugar craving. As the candida dies off, the person will experience serious sugar craving. All sugar alcohols such as Xylitol, maltitol, and glycerol feed candida though to a much smaller extent than regular sugar. Instead, use stevia, a herb that is two hundred times sweeter than sugar, or Guo Han Luo, a fruit from China that is sweet without adversely affecting blood sugar.[9]

After reading all this, treating candida naturally may seem extremely complicated, especially when only one medicine is usually needed in conventional treatment. Nystatin and fluconazole are both very effective conventional drugs. However, in AS because there is often impaired liver function, the fluconazole warning to monitor the liver is of concern. Nystatin works well, but the infections routinely come back as the symptoms, not the cause, is addressed. Natural medicine addresses the cause and if done correctly, should stop future reoccurrences of candida. All these natural substances are aiding in the overall health of the person because they contain beneficial nutrients. And, by withdrawing sugar from the diet, the person sees the connection between eating too much sugar and the candida symptoms.

HYPOGLYCEMIA

Hypoglycemia, a state in which blood glucose drops to below normal levels, seems to be very common in the AS population. This is probably related to the poorly functioning digestive system, especially the ability to digest protein. Most often the person will complain of having increased anxiety and irritability in mid-morning or mid-to-late afternoon. They also always seem to crave sugar or simple carbohydrates. While it can vary in severity, it is easy to control in most people. Start each day with a protein breakfast and eat protein every three to four hours throughout the day. All carbohydrates, whether simple like a cup of coffee with sugar or complex like a bowl of oatmeal, should be accompanied by some form of protein. Taking 400 IU (international units) of chromium is also helpful. Since hypoglycemia is food-related, it will be discussed in greater detail in Chapter 7, the chapter on AS and the impact of diet.

IRRITABLE BOWEL SYNDROME

The bowel is the large intestine in which the body makes and stores stool. When the digestive process isn't working well, the bowel becomes irritated and the person develops symptoms such as constipation, diarrhea, bloating, and gas. There are little to no changes in the walls of the intestines, so it is not considered a disease, but rather a functional disorder. It's also considered a stress-related condition, as it seems to occur more often in anxious people. Though irritable bowel is very uncomfortable, most often it can be treated successfully and quickly. If the main symptoms of the IBS in a child is diarrhea, then check for gluten intolerance.

The best treatment is to rule out food allergies/sensitivities, eat a good diet, take enzymes and probiotics to stabilize the digestive tract, and work on decreasing your stress levels. Most people will need a balance of ten to twenty-five billion units of probiotics two times daily on an empty stomach. Follow the directions on the refrigerated powder for children. We've already covered how to choose a good enzyme. If you aren't sure which part of your digestion seems impaired, then take a broad-based combination of good quality enzymes that will address all the aspects of digestion. Please don't purchase a discount product as they are often poor quality and may not help. We will discuss what a good diet means in great detail in the next chapter.

OTHER DIGESTIVE CONDITIONS

If not adequately addressed, the previously mentioned conditions can develop into more serious conditions such as colitis, diverticulitis or diverticulosis, Crohn's disease, or inflammatory bowel disease. These are beyond the scope of this book. Again, please find a naturopathic or other type of holistic physician to help address these before having any intestines removed. That should be the last resort as it's irreversible. Every part of the intestines has a purpose; none are expendable. Removing parts of the intestines often results in changing one problem for another.

BEYOND THE GUT

Though the digestive tract is most frequently affected in people with AS, there are also a host of seemingly unrelated problems that are routinely seen. In children, there seem to be a higher than normal incidence of headaches and bedwetting. There doesn't seem to be a pattern with the headaches as they occur in the top, back, and sides of the head. I have just noticed that they occur much more commonly in AS children than in non-AS children. I most successfully treat these with homeopathy, which will be discussed in Chapter 10 and changes in the diet in Chapter 7. The bedwetting or enuresis can be related to a host of things including food allergies/sensitivities, food colorings or additives, and inadequate nutrition from a poor quality diet. It is rarely an organic problem such as the size of the child's bladder. Punishing or embarrassing a child with AS for bedwetting is much less effective. No one chooses to wet the bed. Instead, keep a journal of the food or circumstances of the day prior to each episode. If it is a daily occurrence, consider removing the food that the child craves the most and eats daily for a month to see if that is the culprit. Otherwise, look at the recommendations in the following chapter on food allergies/sensitivities.

In AS adults, it's common to see high blood pressure and other heart-related conditions. This is most likely related to the prolonged state of anxiety. Multiple articles by scientists have reported this. For example, a 2006 study by Hungarian researcher Csaba succinctly reported, "Anxiety itself, and anxiety disorders in particular, seem to represent an independent risk factor for cardiovascular diseases as important as obesity, hypertension (high blood pressure), sedentary lifestyle or hyperlipidemia (excessive fatty substances in the blood)."[10] An article by Uyarel et al. confirmed in a study of 726 young men, an association between sudden and prolonged anxiety with irregularities on the ECG heart test.[11] An Australian study by Esler et al. similarly makes the connection between the emotion of anxiety and the physical consequence of heart disease.[12] As with digestive concerns, cardiac health improves as the mental and emotional state of AS becomes more balanced.

SLEEP

Sleep is a frequent issue in both children and adults with AS. Sleep issues include difficulty falling asleep, staying asleep, or waking too early. This is most often related to difficulty in turning off the anxiety and will be addressed in more detail in Chapters 9 and 10. There are many herbs, nutrients, and homeopathic remedies that can help considerably.

TICS AND TOURETTE'S SYNDROME

Another common problem that show up in AS children and often extend into adulthood are tics. Tics can be simple or complex. Examples of simple tics that involve a minimal amount of muscles are blinking, shoulder shrugs, facial grimacing or twitching, head or shoulder jerking, sniffing, throat clearing, grunting, or barking sounds. Complex tics involve several muscle groups and may include a combination of the simple tics. For example, sniffing and shoulder shrugs, or saying a phrase, or hitting oneself in the face. Many times, there is also a family history of Tourette Syndrome, which is a genetic condition commonly associated with OCD (obsessive compulsive disorder), ADHD (attention deficit hyperactivity disorder), dyslexia, depression, sleep dysfunction, and anxiety-related disorders. Persons are diagnosed with Tourette's if they have both vocal and motor tics for at least one year with the onset starting by the age of eighteen. When there is Tourette's in the family tree, the daughter may get OCD-like behavior while the son may manifest the tics. Sometimes tics can be internal. One child described a sensation of "his brain flapping in his head" when he became frustrated. Tics and Tourette's are worse in anxiety-provoking situations and better in calm conditions. If you or your children have these "tics," then all the recommendations in the next few chapters will help considerably.

CHAPTER 7

What You Eat Affects How You Act

One of the least expensive and most effective ways to treat Asperger Syndrome (AS) is with changes in the diet. Improving the quality of food, adjusting the time it is eaten, and avoiding certain foods all help to decrease the intensity of AS symptoms.

At thirty-five, Judy rarely cooked dinner, but preferred to eat out with her husband at dinner or mother at lunch. Though she was on several medications to control her AS symptoms of obsessive-compulsive behavior, extreme anxiety and depression, she was by her own admission, not doing well. But when we recommended organic foods, cooking five dinners at home that included mostly unsaturated fats, protein, and complex carbohydrates, eating two vegetables a day, stopping all desserts, and avoiding all fast foods and processed foods, she gasped. "I can't do all that work. And it will cost way too much." We coaxed her to try it for one month and to reevaluate at that point. Judy e-mailed daily with questions and visited the local health food store for the first time. By the end of the month, she called and said, "My husband says I'm so much easier to live with. I actually have moments when I feel really calm." Since she cut back on eating out, it didn't cost more. And her husband, equally happy with Judy's results, was more than willing to continue with the changes.

So why did altering her diet help so much? Fresh, organic, whole foods are full of usable vitamins, minerals, enzymes, and other nutrients, which are required for mental and emotional balance. In AS, good nutrition calms an overstimulated nervous system, improves focus, and decreases anxiety, overreactivity, and agitation. It also supports the digestive system and helps with liver function, including detoxification. This is especially important because both scientific literature and clinical experience demonstrate that digestive problems and poor liver detoxification are common occurrences in the AS population. In order to better understand what good nutrition means, we can start with defining organic whole foods.

Whole foods are foods in their original form, or very close to it. For example, all fruits and vegetables are whole foods. Meat, poultry, fish, nuts, grains, and beans are whole foods. Foods like butter, most whole-grain pastas, and tofu are one step away from their original food and are generally still considered whole foods. However, processed foods or foods with additives such as pre-made meals both frozen or from a fast-food restaurant are not. Whole foods provide the nutrients your body, brain, and emotions need to stay stable. But while whole foods are integral to your health, it's also important to eat organic foods. Organic foods contain more antioxidants, including Vitamin C and E, than their conventional counterparts. Insecticides and pesticides routinely put on all conventionally grown plants and in our livestock feed not only don't provide any nutritional benefit to the body, but also place an additional burden on the liver. The liver regards them as toxins and must work hard to remove them. Most AS people have impaired ability to remove these toxins, so they may end up lodged in tissues causing daily mood swings, increased anxiety, or irritability. More importantly, insecticides and pesticides target the nervous system of the insects and pests. There is a residual effect on the human nervous system, which will be discussed in greater detail in Chapter 8. And if you ever compared a fresh organic strawberry to a nonorganic one, you would see why people who eat organic also feel the food tastes better.

If you are feeling overwhelmed with the thought of buying and preparing and yes, even eating whole foods, here is some encouragement to get you started. Think of food as proprietary medicines that address both the symptoms and the underlying cause of the condition. Each group of food, such as fruits, vegetables, whole grains, beans, nuts, seeds, fish, poultry, and meat has a slightly different medical profile and performs a specific role in our health. And, food is such a safe form of medicine that there are virtually no side effects or adverse reactions from mixing with other foods. For example, whole grains such as barley, millet, brown rice, and wheat bran are particularly rich in minerals such as magnesium, phosphorus, and potassium as well as the B-vitamin, niacin. In the context of treating AS, these nutrients all help the nervous system work better. When there is insufficient niacin in the body, it decreases the amount of serotonin that can be produced naturally from foods. Serotonin is not only our body's inborn antidepressant, but also our resident antianxiety medicine. Magnesium (in both animal and human studies) has been shown to decrease depression, anxiety-like, and hyperactive behaviors. One of the ways magnesium helps the nervous system is as a catalyst to help activate the various B-vitamins. The B-vitamins are perhaps the most important nutrients we can obtain from our food for a healthy and steady nervous system. Potassium supports the adrenal glands. This is especially important in AS adults who have depleted their adrenals with years of sustained anxiety. And phosphorus steadies the individual nerve impulses—yet another way to normalize the nervous system. When looking at even one food group's effect on the health of the nervous system, you can see why Judy improved so dramatically in one month. She was feeding her starved nervous system with food that would make it work better. She couldn't have done this without eating whole foods. A cup of enriched white rice contains 13 mg. of magnesium and 179 mg of potassium, while a cup of brown rice contains 172 mg of magnesium and 420 mg of potassium. Similarly, enriched wheat flour, the first ingredient in most breads, contains 28 mg of magnesium and 105 mg of potassium versus whole-wheat flour, which contains 136 mg of magnesium and 444 mg of potassium. The nutritional value is even higher in the more nutritious wheat bran logging in at 279 mg of magnesium and 639 mg of potassium. And this disparity exists in all food categories. Iceberg lettuce contains 250 IU units of Vitamin A, compared to 1456 in romaine lettuce and 5963 in kale. Vitamin A is needed to build healthy intestinal linings, a common weak area for those with AS, and is a potent antioxidant. Antioxidants are one important way that the body neutralizes potentially cell-damaging reactions. In studies of cod liver oil, Vitamin A has been shown to help with increasing the ability to socialize and make eye contact. As you can see, food is more than something to put in our mouths. It's the basic fuel for how well each person functions mentally, emotionally, and physically.

The naturally occurring essential fatty acids in foods such as nuts, flax and sesame seeds, salmon, halibut, snapper, cooked soybeans, raw tofu, all winter squash, and avocadoes are also needed to maintain a healthy nervous system. Extremely well researched, essential fatty acids stabilize impulsive behavior, increase seratonin levels, and have shown effectiveness in treating the AD(H)D component of AS. Vegetables such as kale, mustard greens, cauliflower, and carrots not only supply vitamins and minerals but also support liver detoxification. Most foods, if eaten in a fresh, raw, or lightly cooked state contain sufficient enzymes to help the person digest them. But for the majority of people with AS, their digestion is impaired and this isn't enough. Fresh, uncooked herbs such as parsley, basil, cilantro, dill, and thyme contain a therapeutic amount of enzymes. If eaten on a regular basis they will help the person to both digest and absorb the food. For example, parsley contains abundant amounts of the enzyme carbonic anhydrase. This enzyme stimulates the stomach and pancreas secretions, which in turn helps the digestive process work more efficiently. When you go to a Middle Eastern restaurant, you can tell how effective parsley is in digestion. Along with the customary bean dishes of hummus and foule, the restaurants will serve traditional tabouli, a simple combination of mostly parsley with some minced mint, tomatoes, lemon, and shallots. This isn't there as a garnish, but as a means of helping digest the bean dishes. Different enzymes target different parts of digestion. For example, the enzyme, betagulcanase breaks down grains, lipase breaks down fats, and cellulase breaks down candida. Eating organic foods in their whole natural state means a more emotionally stable child or adult. The bottom line is the more organic whole foods a person with AS eats, the less intense the symptoms, which means fewer overreactions and less anxiety as well as a decreased need for medication or even supplements.

Individual vitamins and minerals are just the start of the supportive effects of organic whole foods. Protein in meats, beans, nuts, seeds, poultry, and fish help balance blood sugar. Balanced blood sugar results in fewer emotional outbursts, moodiness, or overreactivity. Hypoglycemia, a condition in which the blood glucose or sugar is imbalanced and dips below normal levels, results in anxiety, lightheadedness, and disorientation. In a person without AS, it would look like mood swings. But in the AS person who is already anxious and oversensitive to stimuli, it would be much more intense and look more like a meltdown, oppositional behavior, or an inexplicable outburst.

There are two main types of hypoglycemia seen in AS: reactive and fasting. Both forms of hypoglycemia can cause mood swings, anxiety, shakiness, confusion, difficulty in speaking, and over-reactivity. In reactive hypoglycemia, a drop in blood glucose and the subsequent symptoms occur about four hours after eating. That's why many children and adults complain of meltdowns or increased irritability mid-morning or a few hours after their last meal. Though fasting hypoglycemia may have many causes including medications, there may also be a deficiency of the enzymes that control the amount of glucose released from the liver. Normally, a few hours after food is eaten, blood sugar or glucose levels start to drop. The liver secretes glucose in order to maintain healthy blood glucose levels. If the liver doesn't have the enzymes to make this adjustment or if the person has taken certain medications, hypoglycemic symptoms will develop. Hypoglycemia tends to be worse in people who eat a high simple carbohydrate diet and routinely skip meals. The way to avoid this is to eat regular and frequent meals that include protein. For people who get irritable, or are unable to concentrate mid-to-late morning, or find they must have a cup of coffee or a treat at this time, I often suggest eating a more substantial breakfast. And, after changing to a protein breakfast with whole grains such as eggs and whole grain bread or oatmeal with nuts, most patients report back that their earlier symptoms disappeared and their mood and energy stayed balanced.

Twelve-year-old Brian was a typical AS child, very sweet and trusting, but a little-out-of-sync with his classmates. Every day, around 11 a.m. he would be mercilessly teased by a few classmates until he broke down and cried. His therapist and parents suggested strategy after strategy, but nothing helped. When he came to my office, I discovered he routinely ate a popular cereal each morning for breakfast. As part of the treatment plan, I proposed to his mom that she makes him a protein breakfast every morning and to eat a handful of almonds right before the 11 a.m. class. Within a week, the bullies were no longer able to goad him. With his nervous system steadier, he could successfully employ the coping strategies that his therapist and parents recommended. The ten extra minutes Brian's mom spent cooking his breakfast every morning were more than worth the smile on his face and increased self-esteem. Eventually, he even learned how to cook simple breakfasts himself.

SUGAR

A problem similar to hypoglycemia that seems almost universal in the Asperger population is a sensitivity to sugar.

Joe was a shy and sensitive eleven-year-old with Asperger Syndrome. His mother would wryly joke that he could turn into a clawing animal, and usually at the worst and most embarrassing times, such as church and school parties. Imagine a sweet child getting so out of control that he clawed not only through the teacher's shirt, but also scratched her skin. It was very fortunate for him that the teacher was a friend of the family and realized that something was very wrong. On Joe's first visit, we discussed his diet in detail. It was obvious that he was extremely sensitive to sugar. And while this was subsequently confirmed with a test, we decided the case was so extreme that we would remove sugar right away from his diet. Within three days of no sugar, his angry outbursts decreased by 80 percent. One month later, his mom let him go on his first church outing with a strict request for the organizers to not give Joe sugar. A skeptical parent chaperone probably thinking that Joe's mom was being excessive, offered him a cookie. Within a few minutes, he clawed the bewildered parent who hastily called Joe's mom.

After repeating this sugar-free diet in more than a hundred patients, it became clear that this wasn't an isolated reaction. Without exception, they all demonstrated less anxiety and agitation. It was extremely interesting to hear the individual reports on earlier symptoms now decreased or eliminated once sugar was removed. Tom, a twenty-year-old college student learned that his all-day headaches were related to sugar, while Mary, a middle-aged realtor, realized her arthritis was linked to her sweet tooth.

Sugar metabolizes in the brain differently in people with AS than others. There is a decreased ability to metabolize glucose in the brain. That means that glucose, usually a brain fuel, is not processed well by the AS brain. The excess glucose results in overloaded circuits commonly manifesting as hyperactivity and overreactivity. We see this extreme sensitivity to sugar in virtually 99 percent of people with AS. University of California, Los Angeles Professor James Barnard, a well-respected researcher in this area, found that refined sugars harm brains specifically by reducing the function of the hippocampus, neuronal plasticity, and learning.[1] The hippocampus is the part of the brain involved with memory, learning, and emotion. Neuronal plasticity refers to the ability of nerves and neurons to adapt to whatever is going on in daily life such as learning, handling new situations, or even rebounding after emotional reversals. Sugar has also been linked to anxiety and depression. An interesting study in 2002 by Westover et al. from the Baylor College of Medicine in Houston, Texas, found a correlation between the consumption of sugar and the annual rate of major depression when reviewing UN (United Nations) statistics for various countries.[2] A 2001 article in *NeuroReport* by Princeton researchers concluded that excessive sugar binds to opioid receptors in the brain much like some drugs of abuse.[3] Another study showed the correlation between increased stress and anxiety and the desire for sugar.[4] When the subjects were given medication for their anxiety, they had a decreased compulsion to eat sweets. In the clinic, we see an even stronger response to sugar in children. A 1995 Yale study by Jones et al. explained this. They examined the effect of sugar on the nervous system with twenty-five healthy children and twenty-three young healthy adults. They concluded that sugar invoked an even greater stress and anxiety response in children via its effect on the adrenals and contributed to adverse behavior and cognitive function.[5] Researchers Lien and Heyerdalh, reported among a group of 5,498 tenth-graders, a correlation between drinking soft drinks and manifesting hyperactivity, mental distress, and conduct problems.[6] For these reasons, we recommend a complete avoidance of sugar.

When I prescribe removing sugar from the diet, even the most confident patient blanches. The children verbalize this sentiment with either a torrent of complaints or a stony stare. In order to get compliance, I only ask people to remove sugar for one month. With a warning to wait until a weekend, I suggest that at the end of the month the adult or child to eat as much sugar as they want. Most often anxiety or forgotten physical complaints return in full force. Then, we work on determining how much sugar each person can take without worsening the symptoms. The overall goal isn't to remove sugar permanently from the diet, but to clearly see its effect and to discover safe levels that won't trigger a response. Most people can safely tolerate some sugar, about 25 percent can't.

The best way to successfully remove sugar from the diet is when the whole family or household joins in. It's too hard on one family member, especially children, to be the only one not eating desserts, catsup, and barbecued ribs. And because of the genetic component to AS, other family members often have other neurological conditions of their own. For example, most AS patients have siblings or patients with ADD or ADHD. They will similarly benefit from removing sugar. When sugar is taken out of the diet, it needs to be taken out of the house, not just hidden.

Sugar is almost revered in our culture. When I suggest that it be removed from the child's diet, one would think I was suggesting that the parents remove all the child's toys. In fact, what I often see in new patients is that parents have loaded their child up on various B-vitamins and minerals. They are trying to help maintain some control over the child's behavior, but are in reality only compensating for the negative effects of sugar. They will spend for unnecessary pills and then force their child to take them when removing sugar would save them money and aggravation.

While it is using up the body's stores of valuable B-vitamins, sugar also increases the excretion of calcium. Your body maintains specific ratios of minerals to each other. For example, a healthy calcium to magnesium ratio may range from 3:1–2:1. If you don't have enough calcium to maintain this ratio because it has been excreted by sugar, then even with an adequate intake of magnesium, you may find the usable magnesium levels low. The paradox is, you can simultaneously have healthy blood levels of magnesium but are unable to use it efficiently because of the decreased calcium.

People who crave sugar develop "sugar radar." One wife hid the sugar in a plastic bag in the bottom of her laundry hamper; her husband found it by the end of the second day. A two-year-old climbed the cupboard shelves to search for sugar; his mom only found out when he shouted for help to get down. So, all the sugar must be taken out of the house. Give it to a neighbor or relative for safekeeping. One mom put it in the trunk of her car and kept the keys with her. It can't be overstated; the single most effective dietary change a person can make in decreasing the symptoms of AS is removing sugar from the diet. As one mom who had been resisting my sugar recommendation said to me, "If I had known the change would be this rapid and positive, I would have done it immediately. It is more than worth the inconvenience to have a more peaceful home."

In some people, food additives or preservatives act as triggers for emotional outbursts or shutdowns.

Karen is a thirty-one-year-old computer software engineer who was having trouble at work, especially in the afternoon. Even though she ate a very low-sugar diet, and tried to eat protein throughout the day, she would find herself shrinking in her cubicle every afternoon a few hours after lunch. She felt so overwhelmed with anxiety that she could barely deal with anyone. In my office we discussed what she was eating for lunch. She would either get a lunchmeat sandwich or a salad and dressing from a local restaurant. What both these foods have in common are sulfites. While we waited on test results to confirm the sulfite sensitivity, Karen decided to go ahead and bring in organic lunchmeats and her own salads and salad dressing. Within a few days, her after-lunch anxiety had decreased to a manageable level.

Sensitivity to sulfites and food coloring is more common than you would think. My best clue to look for this is when the person's favorite food is hotdogs. Or if the child seems to get agitated after taking his brightly colored multivitamin. There are lab tests that can confirm if the food additive or preservative is contributing to the condition.

Occasionally, a parent will come out and flatly say that her child just won't eat any new foods. Adults are more subtle about it and will make comments like, "I tend to like just a few things." In many of these cases, the AS sensory issue is sensitivity to tastes and/or texture. If the problem is texture, work around that by putting the food in an acceptable texture. Vegetables can be pureed into a soup that is still very nourishing. In taste issues, there may be a zinc deficiency. Too little zinc, a common occurrence in the AS community, may result in altered taste buds. A simple lab test can determine this. A trip to a naturopathic doctor's office for an unofficial zinc tally test will give similar results. It takes about six exposures to a food for the sensitive person to accept a new taste. Expect the food-sensitive child to spit the food out the first few times. I suggest you plan on it so it doesn't surprise you when it happens. Eventually, most new tastes will be assimilated.

When tackling the daunting task of changing the diet, there are two main strategies. Strategy 1 is to slowly incorporate healthier food into the diet. This is a useful strategy to adopt in families where there may be resistance to dietary changes from one of the parents. This strategy will result in gradual but steady improvement over two to three months. In adult AS patients, and those who want more rapid results, Strategy 2, a more aggressive approach, will show dramatic improvement frequently within one week.

Strategy 1: The Gradual Change

The easiest place to start is to increase protein in the diet starting with breakfast. If breakfast is a sugar cereal and juice or coffee, add protein in the form of nuts, eggs, or bacon, or sausage. Another option is the very healthy Central American breakfast of beans and eggs. For some people, even eating breakfast is a challenge. They have gotten into the habit of completely skipping breakfast. They grab a cup of coffee and head out the door. If your stomach isn't ready for solid food, then drink a protein drink instead. Buy an unsweetened protein powder and add half of an organic frozen banana or a half-cup of organic frozen berries in the blender as your sweetener. Gradually, your stomach will acclimate to healthy breakfast foods. Often those who don't eat breakfast eat a huge dinner. Skip dinner for one night and you will definitely be more inclined to eat a good breakfast the next day. Eating a breakfast with protein and whole grains will help keep the mood more stable throughout the day.

Along with a healthy breakfast, protein throughout the day is critical. If you are having a salad for lunch, make sure that it includes some form of protein such as chicken, tofu, eggs, or nuts. If you are sending your AS child to school, substitute a nitrate-free sliced meat sandwich for the peanut butter and jelly. Or if they eat the school lunches, look over the weekly menus and discuss the healthier options. I find that when the child is brought in on the discussion of food, there is much better compliance.

After a steady influx of protein has been added to the diet, replace the all nonorganic foods with their organic counterparts. Some grocery stores and all natural food stores have organic meat. For those who are concerned about cost, there are food co-ops in many areas where in exchange for a few hours of volunteering a month, there is a reduction in food costs.

The next step is to adopt a modified Feingold diet. In the 1960s, Dr. Benjamin Feingold, the Head Physician in the Allergy Department in Kaiser Foundation Hospital in Northern California, was one of the early pioneers in studying nutrition-affected behavior. He advocated removing all synthetic food dyes, artificial flavors, and preservatives from the diet. In addition, he recommended removal of a food group called "natural salicylates." These are foods such as grapes, tomatoes, peaches, cucumbers, almonds, peanuts, and peppers. While I find that many of my patients, like the general population, are sensitive to one or two salicylates, they are not sensitive to them all and it is an unnecessary hardship to remove them all from the diet. What the modified Feingold diet means in terms of your food choices is to avoid 90 percent of all processed foods and fast foods. Read the labels. If you initially need processed foods for emergency meals, look for the health food store variation. But please take out all food colorings including those found in children's vitamins. The significance of food coloring and additives will be discussed in greater detail in Chapter 9.

Removing Sugar from the Diet

The next huge challenge is removing sugar. Many people say that they don't eat a lot of sugar—until they look at virtually every processed food they routinely buy. Sugar is in everything: catsup, pastries, cookies, and other sweets; beverages—sodas, juices, punch, dried fruits, fruit leathers, fruit, many sauces such as barbecue sauce and salad dressings, fruit-flavored yogurt, frozen yogurt, donuts, muffins, fruit-sugar drinks, juice bars, energy bars (except a few that are sweetened with glycerin or alcohol sugars like maltitol), jam, jelly, most popular brands of peanut butter, gum, hot cocoa, ice-tea, tapioca, sweetened tea, sweetened breakfast cereals (90 percent of the cereal market), pudding, breakfast convenience foods put in the toaster, ice-cream, jello, candy, granola, and many processed food dinner products. Alcohol in any form metabolizes like sugar and is in the same classification.

Making it even more difficult to identify sugar, manufacturers use terms the average consumer might not recognize as sugar:

Brown Rice Syrup	High-fructose Corn Syrup
Brown Sugar	Honey
Cane Juice	Invert Sugar
Cane Sugar	Lactose
Cane anything	Levulose
Confectioners Sugar	Maltose
Corn Sweeteners	Maple Syrup
Cornstarch	Molasses
Dextrose	Raw Sugar
Fructose	Sucanat
Galactose	Sucrose
Glucose	Turbinado
Granulated Sugar	White Sugar

This can be confusing to the person trying to eliminate sugar from the diet. The safest way to be sure of what you are eating is to cook from whole foods.

Sugar has a similar effect to many addictive drugs including withdrawal symptoms.[7] Because of this effect on the brain, sugar can't be eliminated in one day without potential withdrawal symptoms such as headaches, dizziness, fatigue, and some stomach upset. Therefore the best way to start is to eliminate the obvious sugars over the first few days. That way these symptoms can be avoided. Remove candy, table sugar, honey, maple syrup, desserts, sugar cereal, soda, juices, and all sweet treats. Then look for and remove the hidden sugars such as catsup, some popular brands of peanut butter, many salad dressings, and barbecue sauce. Read all labels. The month starts on the first day of no sugar. It's fine to have a pear, one cup of berries, or an apple daily, but for that first month, please avoid all other fruit.

A few of my patients have complained of weakness or fatigue when they stopped eating sugar. They wondered if they could have a deficiency in sugar. Even on a no processed sugar diet, it is virtually impossible and extremely unhealthy to remove all natural sugar from the diet. There are natural sugars in all vegetables, grains, and beans. A cup of broccoli has 91 mg of sucrose and 619 mg of fructose! However, natural sugars like those present in whole foods won't adversely affect the nervous system. The reason for the weakness or fatigue is most commonly hypoglycemia. Not enough protein is being consumed as often as necessary and the person's blood sugar is going below healthy levels. A second reason is the body is adjusting to the lack of the sugar stimulant effect. Sugar cravers often avoid the sugar drop by eating sugar throughout the day. Once they stop, their bodies need a little time to rebalance.

At some point, nearly every patient will ask, "Can I just cut way back on sugar?" The answer is no. It doesn't seem to work just by cutting way back. I always have some skeptical patients who try it and just don't get the same results. Sugar, in people with a tendency toward neurological conditions, literally acts like a drug. Removing sugar is like a detox program; there are no halfway measures.

CAFFEINE

Drinking coffee is a sacred ritual for many adults. It's a reason to sit down with friends and a help to get started in the morning. For people with AS, it can exacerbate many of the symptoms. Few realize that while they are drinking their one to three cups daily, the coffee is depleting their bodies of niacin, potassium, magnesium, and manganese. All of these are needed for a balanced nervous system. For example, low levels of niacin decreases the availability of serotonin, a much-needed neurotransmitter involved with ameliorating depression, anxiety, and obsessive-compulsive behaviors. Because of the high levels of anxiety, people with AS are often in a stressful state in which their adrenals are secreting substantial amounts of cortisol. Caffeine amplifies this state because it raises the level of cortisol in the body. Put another way, caffeine increases the level of anxiety. Prolonged anxiety states make the person with AS more likely to develop hypertension or high blood pressure. Coffee, by feeding the anxiety state through increased levels of cortisol, contributes to high blood pressure. Potassium, magnesium, and manganese, three minerals that coffee depletes are necessary to stabilize the nervous system. Potassium and magnesium are associated with lower blood pressure. How much coffee is too much? I find the best answer to that question is for the person to wean themselves off coffee for two months and then return to it. Usually, after that first cup following the two months, the person realizes just how much the coffee was affecting them and will have a much better basis to make the decision to permanently avoid it.

Many people want to know if tea is any better. Tea is marginally better and can be used to wean the person off coffee. Eventually, only an occasional cup of green tea or decaffeinated coffee is fine.

INTRODUCING VEGETABLES AND WHOLE GRAINS

The next step is adding vegetables and whole grains. In my office, when I discuss kale, chard, and collard greens, many of my patients think I'm talking about rabbit food or decorations on a deli plate. What most people don't realize is that these three are leafy greens, which are good sources of calcium, potassium, vitamin A, and various B-vitamins, all of which work together to support a healthy nervous system. These leafy greens, along with the members of the brassica family (broccoli, cabbage, Brussels sprouts, and cauliflower, etc.) also have various heavy metal detoxifying sulfur compounds, which will be discussed further in Chapter 8. If you are still scratching your head and wondering just how you can eat these foods, look at the list of cookbooks in the Appendix. Some of them are specifically designed to help gently add vegetables to the diet without a family revolt. Some general advice is to mince the greens very finely, and add them to tomato sauce, soups, chilies, and lasagnas. In fact, even in my own household, I have never served a lasagna without greens mixed into the pasta layers. For as any good cook knows, the strength of the lasagna is in the sauce and the quality of the cheeses.

Whole grains are a controversial topic in the Asperger community. It centers on the inability of most autistic people to digest gluten. Gluten is a common protein found in all forms of wheat, rye, oats, barley, kasha, millet, triticale, amaranth, spelt, teff, quinoa, or kamut. I find that roughly 80 percent of autistic people do well with this diet, but only 25 percent of those with AS benefit from it. For the other 75 percent, whole grains are extremely nourishing to the nervous system. So I recommend whole grains such as spelt, quinoa, oats, barley, rye, wild rice, millet, amaranth, and yes, some whole wheat in the diet unless the person clearly does poorly on wheat or gluten. If you are not sure, you can either have your doctor do a lab test for gluten sensitivity (Anti-Gliadin Antibodies (AGA), IgG and IgA) or do a one to three-month trial of eliminating gluten from the diet. If there is a noticeable improvement in anxiety and behavior-control, then you are sensitive to gluten. For the rest, grains are an integral part of maintaining a healthy nervous system.

The Atkins diet clearly demonstrates this point. Despite their weight loss, many who adhered to this diet felt unsettled and irritable while following this grain-free diet. And remember to keep the grains mostly in their whole form with their outer covering intact. That means, try to eat the grains in their natural form and not converted into flour. That doesn't mean that whole grains converted to flours are nutritionally worthless, just that the whole grains are substantially better for you.

Incorporating whole grains into the diet can be tricky. And frankly, when I start talking about whole grains, my patients' eyes gloss over even more than when we discuss vegetables. Here are a few easy ways to start incorporating whole grains into the diet. Eat unprocessed whole grain cereal for your breakfast a few days a week. Bob's Red Mill Brand has several good multigrain breakfast cereals for the winter. Add some fresh blueberries, almonds, cinnamon, and it becomes a very calming way to start the morning. Wild rice is another wonderful addition.

A great way to prepare it is cooked in bouillon and served with sautéed onion, garlic, and little pieces of cooked meat. Add some black pepper, for some added flavor. Cook up some cracked wheat and add to your chili. And when you make muffins, add half a cup of a whole grain such as wheat or rice bran for added nutrition and flavor. Buy the coarser grades of cornmeal for cornmeal muffins. Fortunately, there are preflavored whole grain mixes, which cook up in thirty to sixty minutes. A general rule of thumb with packages of grain products is that if they take under ten minutes to cook, then they are too refined and have marginal nutritional value, which means that they won't do much to lessen AS symptoms.

Along with fresh vegetables and whole grains are fresh herbs such as parsley, basil, oregano, sage, chives, garlic, cilantro, dill, thyme, and rosemary. Each has mild medicinal value. Fresh basil helps with healing and avoiding ulcers as well as neutralizing harmful substances, while fresh parsley clears toxins from the body via the kidneys and because of its antioxidant constituents, is also protective of the liver.[8–10] Dill is traditionally used to help with gas, colic, bad breath, protects the intestinal lining, and is effective against the mold Aspergillus niger, and the yeasts Saccharomyces cerevisiae and Candida albicans.[11, 12] It tastes delicious in potato salad, on a baked potato with the usual fixings or in a creamed soup. The well-researched list of the benefits of garlic includes antiviral, antibacterial, and antifungal properties. Experiment with fresh herbs and then include the ones you like into your diet. Fresh herbs are considered a gourmet's delight and anyone who has tasted a tomato sauce with fresh herbs will certainly agree.

Strategy 1 in Review:

1. Eat proteins throughout the day.
2. Replace all foods with their organic equivalent.
3. Remove all artificial dyes, preservatives, and additives.
4. Remove sugar from the diet.
5. Add vegetables and whole grains to the diet.

Strategy 2—The Aggressive Change

Start with removing sugar from the diet. It can't be repeated enough, removing sugar from the diet is the single most important dietary change you can make in decreasing AS. Most people see the effects within a few days and are willing to then proceed to the other nutritional changes.

Artificial Sweeteners

Often people ask about artificial sweeteners as viable substitutes for sugar. Many consider artificial sugars benign sweeteners that are a step above sugar. Actually, there are many different types of artificial sugars and they fall into varied health categories. The main forms of artificial sweeteners are aspartame, sucralose, saccharin, the alcohol sugars such as Xylitol, maltitol, sorbitol, and glycerol, and the herb stevia.

Aspartame

Aspartame has been on the market for decades and has an interesting safety track record. There are isolated medical journal articles that connect aspartame with fibromyalgia and damage to the brain cells.[13] While there are very few adverse research papers from the scientific journals, there are thousands of anecdotal accounts of adverse reactions ranging from headaches to increased epileptic seizures. This discrepancy suggests either many people are falsely attributing symptoms to aspartame or that insufficient research has been done. More specific to AS, aspartame excites glutamate receptors in the brain. Excessive amount of glutamate adversely affect memory and learning as well as make it tough for people with Asperger Syndrome to calm down. It's best for those with AS to avoid foods with aspartame in it.

Sucralose

Sucralose, also known as Splenda is starting to dominate the artificial sweetener market. Chemically, sucralose is sugar with hydrogen atoms taken off and chlorine atoms added. Twenty percent of all American homes use sucralose in their diet. We have no long-term studies showing its safety—or toxicity. A 2002 mouse study by the Hachinohe National College of Technology in Japan showed sucralose, along with saccharin, induced DNA damage, or potential cancer-forming cell changes, in the digestive tract.[14] Another study, by the McNeil Specialty Products Company, a wholly owned subsidiary of Johnson and Johnson, which produces sweeteners, found kidney abnormalities in all female treatment groups, bleeding in the adrenals in high-dose group female rats, and increased incidence of cataracts in the male rats.[15] There have been very few human trials on the safety of sucralose. The longest study tested the safety of sucralose for thirteen weeks and found no adverse effects.[16] However, similar to aspartame, there are many anecdotal accounts of harm related to sucralose. Dr. Joseph Mercola, a popular Internet medical site lists the following: allergic reactions: drop attacks (psuedostrokes), abdominal cramping, hives, heart palpitations, dizziness, nausea, diarrhea, sleeplessness, and anxiety.[17] For better or worse, over the next twenty years, people who regularly use sucralose will reveal its safety or toxicity. They are the guinea pigs for the sucralose industry. The best advice for the AS population is to avoid artificial sweeteners, but if you want a sucralose-sweetened treat, to eat them in moderation and not daily. If you have unresolved intestinal complaints and you eat sucralose daily, then do a trial of one month avoiding it so you can see if it has any effect on your particular symptoms.

Saccharin

Saccharin has been around for over a hundred years. During this time, dozens of medical studies have confirmed it to be noncarcinogenic in humans. However, there were a few studies in the medical journals that suggested it is not as safe as may have previously been thought. A couple of articles advanced a possible link between the use of saccharin and changes in the cells lining the colon.[18, 19] Going one step further, a study proposed that saccharin is a causative factor for inflammatory bowel disease.[20] Some research proposes a link between excessive use of saccharin and iron and folate deficiencies.[21] Most of these were animal studies and there has been insufficient human research to draw any clear conclusions. In those with AS, the only concern with saccharin is its possible link to intestinal changes. In a population of already weakened digestive health, saccharin use should be minimal.

Sugar Alternatives

Stevia

Stevia rebaudiana is a South American herb, which has spread throughout the world to become a sweetener in Japan, China, India, and parts of Southeast Asia as well as in the United States. It is between 150 and 400 times sweeter than sugar, but can have a metallic aftertaste similar to saccharin. Though traditionally used as a sweetener for diabetics, stevia has been extensively studied since the 1970s. This research has demonstrated its ability to actually treat diabetes because of its blood glucose stabilizing properties. Several studies even suggest its effectiveness in treating high blood pressure.[22–24] There have been no studies linking stevia with cancer. Even though research on stevia is overwhelmingly positive, I don't recommend the use of stevia as a replacement for sugar. Herbs are medicine and should be treated cautiously. However, stevia seems extremely safe in small amounts such as under half a teaspoon daily for the general public.

Sugar Alcohols

Glycerin or glycerol is an alcohol sweetener similar to Xylitol and is commonly found in high protein, low-carb energy bars. Glycerol converts to glucose in the liver and therefore has a minimal effect on blood sugar. Glycerol can help maintain hydration. This includes treating dry skin, keeping athletes well hydrated during sports events, and in treating acute attacks of glaucoma. Except for the fact that glycerol seems to intensify cases of intestinal candida, which is fairly commonplace among people with AS, glycerol seems safe in small amounts.

Xylitol, Maltitol, and Sorbitol, are sugar-alcohol sweeteners frequently found in sugar-free gums, which seem to have some effect on protecting the teeth from developing cavities. More directly related to people with AS, these alcohol sugars have a moderating effect on intestinal candida overgrowth compared to glucose and sucrose, which means, while it doesn't heal candida, it definitely doesn't feed it at the same degree as regular sugars. All sugar alcohols increase the absorption of calcium.[25] While in moderation, this is beneficial; in larger doses, it can cause an imbalance with the other trace minerals in the body potentially resulting in calcium loss. For some, these alcohol sugars may cause flatulence and diarrhea. They are considered very safe and noncarcinogenic.

Luo Han Guo Fruit Syrup

Grown in the mountains of China, Luo Han Guo, *Momordia grosvenorii*, or *Siraitia grosvenorii*, is a unique fruit in that it has a sweet taste without any nutrients in it like glucose or fructose that can adversely affect the nervous system. Traditionally, it is used medicinally to aid healthy elimination and as a natural sweetener for diabetics. There are a few medical studies that are isolating the major components of the fruit to determine how it balances blood sugar, but the mechanism is still not well-defined.[26, 27] It has a mild sweet taste similar to a light honey, no aftertaste, and lends itself easily as a syrup over pancakes or waffles. There are several companies manufacturing this product in the United States. They generally combine Luo Han Guo with a sugar alcohol such as maltitol to increase its sweetness for the Western palate. As demonstration of the fruit's support of the digestive tract, the flatulence that can accompany the use of sugar alcohols is absent. Some of the companies are isolating components and not using the complete fruit. Look for a company using the whole fruit as it has more nutritional and medicinal value. There is a good source listed in the Appendix. The American Food and Drug Administration (FDA) classify this food as a GRAS (generally recognized as safe) product. There is no known toxicity.

Even though eating an organic whole foods diet is important for everyone, in the AS population, it may not be enough. In many cases, absorption and digestion aren't working well enough to utilize all the nutrients in even a very good diet. In those cases, we need to address the functioning of the digestive tract.

We discussed earlier about the digestive tract being a giant tube starting with your mouth and ending with your anus. Each part of this tube has specific roles in the digestive process. For example, the stomach and intestines support healthy digestion by an elaborate system of secretions that break down food and absorb the valuable nutrients in the food that nourish all the different systems in the body including the nervous system. Healthy intestines also have a balance of beneficial bacteria and fungi. This balance can be disrupted by rounds of antibiotics and leave the person vulnerable not only to illness but also to increased AS symptoms. Determining which foods may be provoking AS symptoms and removing those foods is an important step. The person removes the foods, feels better, and thinks the problem is solved. A few months later, the symptoms return and they remove more and more foods. I have seen many patients, often children, who eat less than ten foods for their entire diet. Even worse, several of these foods tend to be processed and of even less nutritional value. It's hard, if not impossible, to eat a well-balanced diet that provides adequate nutrition when eating only ten foods. That limited a diet generally can't provide the right mix of vitamins, minerals, and other nutrients needed for a healthy nervous system. The most effective treatment process is to test to determine which foods trigger the symptoms, remove them for a few months, heal the intestinal lining, and then return these foods to the diet in moderation. If these three processes are done together, there is a much greater likelihood of a more permanent improvement. As a positive secondary effect, while you are healing the intestines, any digestive conditions such as Irritable Bowel Syndrome, stomach and intestinal ulcers, or erosions will also be improving. It will even help with more serious conditions such as Crohn's Disease or colitis.

In order to understand the process, here's an overview of tests, including some free ones, which determine which foods may be affecting your intestinal health. People often go to an allergist to try to figure out which foods may be affecting them. Allergists can determine allergies, but not food sensitivities or food intolerances. A food allergy occurs when a food causes an immunological response to a food. That means the body gets confused and when the food is ingested, it thinks it's a toxin and puts an elaborate defense system to tag, destroy, or neutralize the effect of that food. The important thing to remember is that the body uses immunoglobulin E (IgE) antibodies in this defense. This is pretty rare and occurs in only 1–3 percent of the population. These are those cases in which a person eats a peanut resulting in an anaphylactic reaction and the person needs either a shot of epinephrine or is rushed to the hospital. Another form of food allergy is a delayed response food allergy. The symptoms are less severe and most often don't happen in minutes, but in hours to days. In these cases it is not IgE, but immunoglobulin G (IgG) that is affected. The person has a delayed reaction, which, while not as life-threatening as food allergies, is still serious and can affect the person in a significant way. This delayed reaction is much more common and can occur in 10–20 percent of the population.

People with AS do not appear to have a higher incidence of IgE food allergies, but seem to have increased IgG food sensitivities and other food intolerances than those of the general population. Intolerances are reactions to food in which neither IgE nor IgG is activated. For example, some people with AS lack enzymes to digest dairy or their body reactions to gluten in an IgA immunological response that will differ from an IgE food allergy or IgG food sensitivity. Often conventional tests can't confirm an allergy to that particular food despite the obvious behavioral changes that occur after the person eats the food.

Johnny, an active little three-year-old boy with AS came to my office with multiple concerns including self-injurious behavior. He would routinely hurt himself either by pounding his head against the floor or wall—a behavior that he exhibited with no prompting in my office. He had already been to an allergist and had tested negative for all suspected allergies. Yet this behavior continued. His favorite foods were pretty much anything and everything made from dairy products ranging from macaroni and cheese to ice-cream to even cottage cheese. I wondered if his head pounding was his way of dealing with a sinus headache. We removed dairy products for a month and the head banging decreased by 90 percent.

Johnny wasn't allergic to dairy products, he just didn't produce the correct enzyme to digest it.

FOOD ALLERGY/SENSITIVITY DIAGNOSTIC TESTING METHODS

Conventional allergists are focused on the IgE immediate allergy response, while complementary and alternative physicians are looking for both IgE and IgG reactions. Most doctors rely heavily on one form or another. And while these tests are an effective way to get the patient to comply with dietary changes as a person will have a hard time refuting a lab result, none are 100 percent reliable and each is limited in one way or another. The following is a list of only the main tests.

Allergy Prick Tests—The starting point for most people in figuring out what foods they may be allergic to is in their allergist's office with the Allergy Prick Test. In this test, a small amount of an extract of the possible allergen, in this case the offending food, is introduced into the skin. If a wheal or any other form of raised inflamed skin occurs, then the person is allergic to that food. The skin test is a good indicator of IgE reactions, but not of the more common IgG.

Intradermal Test—Just as the name suggests, a small amount of the food in extract form is injected under the skin. It's more sensitive than the prick test and is often used if the prick test is negative, but the food is still suspected. However, just like the Allergy Prick Tests, the intradermal tests give a reasonable accurate IgE, but not IgG picture of what is happening in the person.

Rast Test—The Rast (radioallerosorbent) Test is a conventional blood test to determine IgE reactions. It's used when there is a history of an anaphylactic reaction or when there is a skin rash. It's considered much more accurate for airborne allergens than food allergens. It is not effective in helping to identify food sensitivities as they are related to IgG reactions.

IgG ELISA Assay—This is a blood test, which provides a more complete picture as it can determine both IgE and IgG reactions. The test is only as good as the lab that performs it. With a good lab, this is a reliable test that is considered about 95 percent accurate. Most often this is a blood draw, though some labs do a finger prick test with results consistent to the blood draws. The price of these tests range from $130 (finger prick) to $800 to test for 75–125 foods. Contact information for reputable labs is in the Appendix.

Electrodermal Tests—A noninvasive and painless test that measures variations in the normal electrical current, electrodermal testing was developed by Dr. Reinhold Voll in the late 1950s in Germany, and has been used in Europe for about forty years and in the United States for about twenty years. The patient holds a negative electrode in one hand while the positive probe is placed over an acupuncture point. A potential food allergen is then added to the electrical circuit. Theoretically, a change above the normal range on the galvanometer signifies an increased reaction to the food being screened. This form of testing is not consistently reproducible and therefore has not fared well under scientific scrutiny. I have used this form of testing with some patients and found it reasonably reliable in identifying foods that once removed from the diet, made the patient feel better. It is considered to be about 85 percent accurate for determining food sensitivities.

The basic electrodermal test shouldn't be confused with the host of subsequent generations of diagnostic and treatment computers currently available. In addition to identifying food sensitivities, these machines also claim to treat and eliminate the tendency for the food sensitivity. Again, there is no well-documented research supporting the use of these machines. In a computer dominated age, these products appeal to consumers who want a quick and easy way to identify and treat food-related symptoms. And while it is easy to be incredulous about these types of products, the consumers tend to weed out what works and what doesn't. And so far the market has continued to grow. These second-generation electrodermal tests are marketed under various names such as Accupath 1000, BEST, Biotron, Computron, Dermatron, DiagnoMètre, Eclosion, Elast, Interro, LISTEN System, MORA, Natrix Physiofeedback System, Omega AcuBase, OmegaVision, Orion System, Prophyle, Punctos III, Quantum, and Vitel 618. Use the results of these tests simply as markers. They have had insufficient time and research to really determine their effectiveness.

Four Free Testing Methods

Pulse Test—Here is a free old-fashioned test that is fairly reliable on giving the person a general idea of whether a food affects them. On an empty stomach, take your pulse to determine your average heartrate. Then eat a sample of the food in question. Retest the pulse rate. If the rate increases by at least ten to sixteen beats per minute, then you have very likely identified a food sensitivity. However, it's important that only an isolated food is tested. For example, eat only a piece of cheese not cheese and crackers, or some plain cream, or wheat cereal without milk or sugar. If you eat a slice of bread and your pulse increases, it won't be clear if you are reacting to the wheat, yeast, sweetener, or another ingredient. There are no studies supporting or refuting the reliability of this test.

Elimination Test—This is a test that is accepted by both conventional and natural medical doctors. As the name suggests, the suspected food or foods are eliminated from the diet for one month. If there is an improvement, then that food or foods are confirmed as allergens for that person.

Food Challenge Test—A variation on the elimination diet, the food challenge diet has two main versions. In the first, the person avoids the food

for four to six weeks as with an elimination diet. Then the food is rein-
troduced to determine if there is a reaction. The second version is used
if the person is healthy and if faster results are desired, the person fasts
for three days, and then introduces the suspected food again looking for
a reaction. The fasting version requires the supervision of a physician.

Diet Diary—A mainstay in the alternative medicine community, the diet
diary consists of writing down all that is eaten along with any physical
or mental/emotional symptoms that might occur. Sometimes the pattern
is very obvious, other times a natural medicine physician can determine
the pattern.

Discovering food sensitivities and intolerances can be difficult and is best
accomplished with the help of a physician trained in these kinds of tests. Just be
aware that there can be false negatives and positives with all the lab tests. One
thing I have learned from my patients is that they are invariably correct about
their hunches on what foods affect them—with or without lab confirmation. Lab
tests are a good tool when the person is reacting to multiple foods or as a guide to
start the process. Most importantly, trust what you are feeling in your own body or
what you are seeing in your child's behavior and how it relates to food. Perceptive
moms will tell me that their unborn babies kicked violently in the womb when
they ate certain foods but seemed calm when they avoided the same foods.

Healing the Gut

We've discussed diet and how to recognize which foods may be affecting
the intestines. However, just removing the foods isn't enough. Think of your
intestines as a surface that is being irritated daily by foods that inflame and cause
some erosions to this surface, like using a scrub brush on your dining room table.
Just applying a little polish isn't going to remove the scratches. You need to stop
scrubbing it, then sand it down, make it level again and then put on the furniture
polish. With your intestines, you remove the foods and at the same time heal the
erosions. That way, you are repairing the intestinal walls. If these two processes
are done together, the person, after a few months of avoiding the food, can go
onto eating it again in moderation. If they aren't done together, the person can
start a downward spiral of removing more and more foods from the diet. There are
many supplements and herbs, which help maintain a healthy intestinal balance,
support digestion, and heal intestines battered by less-than-optimal food choices.

Healing Herbs

While you are avoiding foods that irritate the intestinal lining, and replenishing the beneficial bacteria that naturally occurs in your intestines, I suggest
that you speed the process along with herbs that heal the intestinal lining and
support healthy digestion. Herbs that work well together and that are fairly easy

to find are Calendula (*Calendula officinalis*), fennel (*Feoniculum vulgare*), marsh-mallow (*Althea officinalis*) and licorice (*Glycerrhiza glabra*). Each of these herbs have specific medicinal properties, which, when blended, help heal the intestines. Calendula, the common marigold, is well-known for its antiinflammatory and ep-ithelial (internal and external surface cells) healing properties, which means it calms and repairs the damage to the intestinal walls.[28–30] Marshmallow, the plant, not the candy, is not only healing to the intestinal tract but also stimulates the body to produce more friendly bacteria.[31] Both Calendula and *Althea* have an-tioxidant qualities to neutralize any harmful free radicals, which are roaming and highly reactive chemicals causing damage to the intestinal walls.[32, 33] *Althea* and Licorice, similar to Calendula, are also demulcents and soothe, protect, and de-crease irritations of the inflamed intestinal walls.[34] Fennel or *Foeniculum vulgare* minimizes flatulence and bloating and kills some harmful intestinal bacteria.[35] It also helps treat ulcers. If you think of intestinal irritation as the ulcer's kid brother, you can see how fennel would be helpful as well. Calendula and Fennel are both antispasmodics and relax the intestinal muscles.[36] The tea can be made from one tablespoon dry herb per one cup hot water. It should steep for twenty minutes. My patients advised me that it works best in a French press, a cylindrical glass container with a strainer on top commonly used for coffee. I often prescribe quarter cup of the tea or quarter teaspoon of the herbal tincture for children and half teaspoon of the herbal tincture for adults to be taken at the end of each meal. Though this is a very pleasant tasting tea or herbal tincture, some prefer a similar formula in powder form, which they take in a fruit smoothie. When purchasing herbs, make sure they are organic or wild crafted. There are many more herbs, which also repair the intestines, but these are a good place to start.

Glutamine is an amino acid, abundant throughout the body, which maintains the intestinal walls' integrity and function. It helps to moderate what gets past the intestinal walls. Effective in treating ulcers, glutamine is antiinflammatory and is especially beneficial in those with sugar and carbohydrate cravings. Despite its benefits, I tend to be wary of this supplement because it can convert to glutamate, an amino acid that is excitatory to the brain. Think of glutamate as an accelerator to the nervous system. Most people with AS would prefer to decelerate their nervous systems. People with strong ADD-like symptoms without hyperactivity may benefit from it. Those with any sort of hyperactivity may want to avoid it or use it only in combination with herbs and other nutrients.

Probiotics

Once the intestinal lining starts to heal, the beneficial bacteria need to be repopulated. One of the most important supplements in reestablishing a healthy intestinal flora balance are probiotics. As we discussed in Chapter 6, probiotics are strains of friendly bacteria that normally inhabit the intestines but through poor diet or use of antibiotics are no longer in the correct balance or as numerous as is needed. Probiotics support a healthy immune system by limiting the number of harmful bacteria that cause disease and by increasing white blood cells. They secrete enzymes that help break down food. Probiotics have been shown to help with irritable bowel syndrome (IBS) and Crohn's disease, as decreased beneficial bacteria is a factor in both conditions.[37] Over time, probiotics reduce food sensitivities.

Most people recognize the single probiotic bacterial strain, *acidophilus bifidus*. This is just one of dozens of the friendly bacteria that your intestines need to rebalance. I recommend purchasing a probiotic that has at least six to ten different beneficial bacterial strains. The average adult needs at least twenty billion microorganisms daily, while the child aged four and over will do well with five billion microorganisms daily. In a few cases, people get diarrhea after starting probiotics. All that means is that you are starting too aggressively. Stop for a day and then start up again on a lower amount and work up to the full dose. Look for probiotics in the refrigerated section of the health food store or health food area of your supermarket. When you look at the label for the number and quantity of probiotics, check the list of other ingredients. Good quality probiotics don't have additives or preservatives. There are unrefrigerated probiotics, but I don't recommend them except for traveling as they are less stable and consistent in their dosage. Probiotics need to be taken daily on an empty stomach for one to three months depending on the severity of the condition. Even if you feel better in a couple of weeks, it often takes longer to make a more permanent improvement.

Enzymes

Earlier in the chapter, we mentioned Johnny and his inability to digest dairy products due to the lack of enzymes to break it down. This is fairly common in people with AS. Children may report stomachaches, or have diarrhea, or constipation. If they are too young to communicate well, then see if there is acting out after meals. They may be uncomfortable or in real distress and have no way to tell you. Adult patients often mention uncomfortable fullness after a meal, excessive flatulence or burping, and stools that float in the toilet. Others complain of heartburn or more serious intestinal conditions such as IBS, Crohn's Disease, or colitis. If you or your child have these intestinal health concerns, then consider these symptoms as indicators that digestive enzymes are needed. Digestive enzymes help break down food. The four main types are lipase, protease, cellulase, and amylase. Lipase enzymes break down fat, protease enzymes, protein, cellulase enzymes, fiber, and amylase enzymes, carbohydrate.

Raw foods are a good source of enzymes. But in most cases, they only break down the particular food that is being eaten. Eating a raw carrot along with a hamburger won't help your digestive system break down the hamburger. As was mentioned in Chapter 7, eating raw herbs such as parsley and mint will provide enzymes to break down a part of the rest of the meal. But since most people, including those with AS, don't eat raw herbs on a regular basis, digestive enzymes are often needed.

Looking for enzymes in your local health food store can be a daunting prospect. There are so many to choose from. First remember the basics. Consider only products that don't contain fillers. Then consider what the main problem is and get the appropriate enzyme. Review the enzyme section in the last chapter for additional help. If you have trouble with wheat and other carbohydrates, look for a combination of amylase, a protease blend, and glycoamylase. Some wheat-tolerant people find that they can eat wheat products in moderation as long as they take these enzymes. Digestive enzymes should be taken initially with each meal and then gradually weaned down to only heavy meals. I have included some excellent enzyme companies in the Appendix.

Another important reason to use enzymes is to digest pills until your own digestive tract is healthy enough to do that job again.

Scott, a young man with AS, felt his anxiety was taking over his life. He had started out well, had a good job, but soon found himself incapacitated with anxiety. So much so that he was thinking of taking a leave of absence. He came to my office for an alternative to conventional medications. For many years, he watched his mom's dependency on Xanax and was determined not to follow in her footsteps. I removed sugar and gave him a very effective supplement, which I have used successfully in hundreds of people to treat anxiety. The problem was it did nothing. He increased the dose and it helped marginally. We opened the capsules with a little more success. Frustrated, I wondered why he didn't seem to absorb it. We decided to use a high quality enzyme with each dose. That worked. He started to absorb the pills, his anxiety dropped, and he felt more in control. I referred him to a coach specializing in AS adults for additional support.

After foods identified as allergens are removed from the diet and you've treated the digestive tract, we should consider another very important area affecting those with AS—environmental toxins, their effect on the liver, and how to support the liver.

CHAPTER 8

How the Environment Affects Asperger Syndrome

One of the most frustrating things for people about Asperger Syndrome (AS) is that there are so many contributing factors. In about 25–30 percent of my AS patients, even after incorporating a better diet, a multivitamin, a few supplements, and some stress-releasing exercises, there may be other factors, which still intensify AS characteristics such as anxiety and overreactivity. In those cases, I start looking for environmental factors in the home, school, or office, including food, water, and air quality and even in their backyards. These factors include insecticides, pesticides, food additives and preservatives, mold accumulation, fluorescent lights, poor response to vaccinations, tap water, air fresheners, and heavy metal exposure. Once we've identified any substance that may be worsening the symptoms, and either removed or counteracted it, the remaining AS symptoms decrease even further.

Environmental toxicity is becoming an increasingly more serious problem for the general public, but especially for those with conditions that affect the nervous system such as AS. The toxic effects of many of these common environmental chemicals and metals look similar to AS characteristics such as overreactivity, irritability, sleep issues, memory dysfunction, and anxiety. And just like AS, environmental toxicity can affect more than just the nervous system. Asthma, hay fever and itchy skin, headaches, fatigue, hyperactivity, pain in muscles, legs, or joints, persistent bowel problems, halitosis, congestion, irritating twitches, leg-wiggling, depression, mood changes, and brain fog are frequent signs of environmental toxicity.

The scientific community has various names for environmental toxicity including multiple chemical sensitivity (MCS) and Environmental Illness (EI), but they are essentially talking about the same thing, toxic and nontoxic chemical substances in the environment that in sufficient quantities result in unwanted symptoms. Like AS, EI is a continuum of mild to severe cases. Some people may get headaches and anxiety and others are so affected that they must live in sterile environments. And while each condition is a separate and distinct diagnosis, a person may have both AS and EI.

With so many overlapping symptoms, it can be unclear as to what is AS and what are adverse reactions to the environment. One way is to look for mood and physical changes that occur only in one place. For example, there may be increased anxiety or agitation at home or in a room with a new piece of furniture. One of my patients became increasingly anxious each night when watching television. When nothing seemed to help, I asked about possible environmental causes. Her granddaughter had purchased a comforter for her, which had never been washed. The "new clothes" chemicals, especially formaldehyde caused the anxiety. Just for good measure, I asked her to run it through the washing machine two times, and sure enough, her anxiety decreased.

Some people with AS are less in touch with mood changes. For them it may be easier to observe physical changes such as headaches, constant clearing of the throat, or a tightness in the throat. Children often reflect their mental and emotional function through their handwriting and drawing. Comparing a child's handwriting or drawing in several locations will help determine if one of these locations is adversely affecting the child. The same technique can be used after eating suspect additives, preservatives, and chemicals in foods. If you suspect food coloring, have your young child write their name, then eat the food with coloring, and write their name ten minutes later. For adults, it's also helpful to journal moods and diet.

Another simple way to determine sensitivity to a substance, which was discussed in Chapter 7, is checking the pulse rate. Once an average resting pulse rate has been established, any substance that increases the pulse by twenty or more beats should be questioned. One person became dizzy when simply opening a box of fertilizer. Curious to see if her pulse really changed, she tested it and found that it shot up by thirty points.

Environmental influences on children can look different than with adults. In younger children, you may see excessive whining, clinging, repeating same phrases (not autistic echolalia), removing clothing, and/or withdrawal. EI can even look like Tourette's. In adults, it's more often increased anxiety and irritability. Finally, check to see if the symptoms are better on vacation or on weekends.

EI is so varied that in order to give you an idea of what this may look like, this chapter depicts patients with both AS and EI, outlines the research, profiles the more AS-relevant sources of environmental toxicity, describes tests to determine if the toxicity exists, and reviews many current methods to remove the toxins.

Scientists have been studying the effects of environmental toxicity in humans for decades. As with any relatively new area of research, a few independent scientists initiate the research and discussion and then several years later, the federal government analyzes the research and makes a statement as to the effect and safety of the substances. In a U.S. FDA report entitled, "Neurotoxicity: Identifying and Controlling Poisons of the Nervous System," they state "The known or suspected

causes of brain-related disorders include exposures to chemicals such as therapeutic drugs, food additives, foods, cosmetic ingredients, pesticides, and naturally
occurring substances."[1] In 1996, Doris Rapp, an allergist turned environmental
medical physician, wrote a groundbreaking book on environmental toxins in the
school entitled, *Is This Your Child's World?*[2] Over a decade later, it remains as
current as when it was written. Dr. Rapp gives example after example of children
struggling in school because of environmental toxins. It's an eye-opening book
that offers scientific evidence of environmental toxins for behaviors common in
AS but often labeled as AD(H)D (attention deficit hyperactivity disorder), OCD
(obsessive compulsive disorder) and ODD (oppositional defiant disorder).

Recognizing Environmental Illness in a person with AS can be tricky. Signs
that suggest environmental factors are puffy eyes, dark circles under the eyes,
mood changes, mental function, headaches, or stomachaches worsening in some
settings and not others. For example, a teacher or student may feel increased
anxiety in one classroom versus another and then be much better at home.
Some may become symptomatic in the garden supply section of home improvement stores. People with AS maybe more susceptible to EI because of
impaired liver function. Numerous studies by researchers such as Koroly Horvath, Jay Perman, BI Cohen, and Andrew Wakefield demonstrated consistent
findings of impaired liver function in conditions on the autism spectrum, including AS.[3–5]

HOW THE BODY DETOXES

For most people, the liver along with the kidney, intestines, and lungs, routinely
detoxifies these environmental toxins. This process is done in two steps. In the
first, the substance is converted into a secondary substance to be excreted, and
in the second step, this hybrid substance is excreted. With many environmental
toxins the secondary substance may be equally or not more toxic than the original
chemical, as occurs with mercury derivatives including thimerosol. If there is a
delay in excreting this secondary substance, it will circulate in the body and very
often adversely affect the nervous system.

People with AS have an impaired ability for the liver to remove everyday
toxins. If the liver can't break down and excrete the toxin, it lodges in various
places in the body including the brain. This means that exposure to substances
considered harmless to others, may cause anger, irritability, or increased anxiety
in someone with AS. Consider the following example.

Stan was a sweet but occasionally scary little five-year-old boy with AS.
His behavior was unpredictable or so his parents and teacher thought. He
would suddenly get angry and irritable and hit the other children, usually
completely unprovoked. One time, when his teacher asked him to calm
down, he threw the toy he had in his hand and hit her in the face. When
I saw him in my office, it was hard to believe that he was capable of
intimidating an entire class including the teacher. We discussed his diet,

which seemed pretty good. His mom limited how much sugar he consumed, and he ate fruits and vegetables on a regular basis. In fact, he loved dried apricots. His lunch was fine as well. He brought a cold-cut sandwich on whole wheat bread, a piece of fruit, and a bag of a healthier brand of potato chips, and water. The only real concern I had about his diet was that it wasn't organic. I wondered if he wasn't sensitive to the insecticides, pesticides, sulfites, nitrates, or one of the other chemicals routinely added to nonorganic food. A quick lab test showed yes, he was sensitive to sulfites and nitrates. Within one week of replacing the dried apricots and the lunchmeat with their organic counterparts, he was noticeably better. He no longer hit the other children or the teacher and within a month, was no longer considered the class bully.

TOXINS IN OUR FOOD

Dr. Benjamin Feingold, a pediatric allergist in the late 1960s, recognized the impact of insecticides, pesticides, and various additives had on behavior. Based on his work and additional research, I recommend a Feingold-like diet by eating an organic whole foods diet with no additives such as food coloring, artificial flavorings, and all chemical preservatives. I also advise avoiding sugar and nitrates other than what is present in the soil. The Feingold diet suggests an avoidance of salicylates, an extremely common compound found naturally in many foods including apples, grapes, peaches, cucumbers, almonds, or peppers. And while some people may be sensitive to this substance, I find this is pretty rare and don't recommend removal of these foods without testing.

Similarly, some researchers such as Dr. Abram Ber, associate phenolic compounds with neurological disorders linked with AS including OCD.[6] Common phenolic compounds are gallic acid, malvin, pyrrole, serotonin, and norepinephrine. Gallic acid occurs in about 70 percent of all foods including chocolate, walnuts, apples and citrus juices, and green tea, as well as acetaminophen and grape fruit seed extract. Dr. Ber suggests that these gallic acid-containing foods may worsen intestinal permeability. However, USDA (United States Department of Agriculture) reports that gallic acid-containing foods help minimize fungal growth.[7] And since fungal infections are fairly common in the AS population, I tell my patients that if they suspect a sensitivity to these foods, then avoid them, but not to automatically remove many nutritious foods from their diet. Because the autism epidemic has spurred a lot of research, scientists will explore possible causes and solutions for those on the autism spectrum. Some of them will be extremely helpful while others less so. I enthusiastically encourage people to eat a diverse diet of organic whole foods, and educate people on the potential harm of chemical-laced conventional foods.

Nonorganic foods contain a multitude of pesticides that can intensify the symptoms of AS. For example, according to the EPA (Environmental Protection Agency), the insecticide lindane, which is routinely used on children and adults to treat lice, as well as on barley, corn, oats, rye, sorghum, and wheat seeds, can cause damage or destroy nerve tissue.[8] Insecticides and pesticides are engineered to target the nervous system of the insect or pest in the field. These same substances affect the human nervous system as well.[9] They often target neurotransmitters such as dopamine and serotonin. Dopamine is involved with attention, motivation, and memory; while serotonin affects anxiety and mood. This is especially serious in a neurological condition like AS. A 1990 government study reported that insecticides and pesticides affect intellectual functioning, academic skills, abstraction, flexibility of thought, and motor skills; memory disturbances and inability to focus attention; deficits in intelligence, reaction time and manual dexterity; and reduced perceptual speed, increased anxiety, and emotional problems.[10] Organophosphates and carbamate insecticides, two common categories of agricultural chemicals commonly sprayed on our foods affect acetylcholine, a neurotransmitter directly involved with memory and behavior. These substances target brain functions, which are especially compromised in those with AS. And if you consider that exposure of these toxins to children up to six years of age are 2.4 times more than adults,[11] it offers one explanation why AS children often seem more impaired than their AS parents. The United States Congressional Office of Technology Assessment, a nonpartisan analytical agency who analyzed scientific and technical issues for the congress, stated, "In general, [human health] research demonstrates that pesticide poisoning can lead to poor performance is pronounced."[12]

Maleic hydrazide is routinely sprayed on potato crops up to one week before harvesting both as an herbicide and to keep the potato from sprouting. But, in the human body, this chemical blocks seratonin productions by inhibiting the action of vitamin B-6. In just one bag of potato chips or one serving of fast food French Fries or potato chips, there is sufficient maleic hydrazide to significantly deplete the B-6 in your body. I commonly see new patients taking megadoses of B-6 to help their AS. While some B-6 may be necessary, it would be better and cheaper to just avoid the substances that deplete B-6 and other nutrients. The government's position is that there is insignificant amount of residual chemicals in the individual foods. And yes, if we all ate one portion of one food daily this would not pose a problem. But we are all different sizes, in varying states of health, and eat different amounts. The cumulative effect can be significant on the nervous system. There are numerous studies on the adverse effect of insecticides and pesticides on brain function.[13]

Nitrates are most commonly found in cured meats such bacon, sausage, hot dogs and lunchmeats, and drinking water. A 1999 animal study by Porter et al. proposed that nitrates found in drinking water alone may lead to aggressive behavior.[14] The additive effect of nitrates in bacon for breakfast, a hotdog at lunch, and tap water all day has yet to be researched. Yet, when we take them out of the diet, the AS person seems more stable.

Food coloring agents are less well studied for their neurological effects, but are equally problematic. Food coloring agents occur not only in the brightly colored cereals and cake decorations, but also in hamburgers, hotdogs, bologna, cherries, some citrus fruits, some butters and margarines, and fruit juices. Food coloring seems to affect the majority of my AS patients.

If you are uncertain if it is affecting your child, have them draw a picture or write their name before and fifteen to thirty minutes after eating a food that has been artificially colored. If there is no change, then they are fine with that particular color. With adults that doesn't work so well. In adults, it's better to do the pulse test and see if there is a twenty or more increase in pulse rate. Routinely, after a month of only organic foods, patients report less anxiety and less outbursts and feelings of being overwhelmed. There are lab tests, which I will outline later in the chapter, which will determine if you have high levels of chemical toxins in your system.

But organic foods are not just important for what they don't have, but for what they do have. Multiple independent studies conclude vitamin C and E and beta-carotene were consistently higher in organic versus nonorganic fruit and vegetables.[15–18] Phenolic compounds such as bioflavonoids, are naturally occurring plant substances that possess antioxidant and antiinflammatory properties. This becomes more significant when you consider the intestinal inflammation that regularly accompanies AS. As a University of California-Davis study by Asami, Mitchell et al. published in 2003 demonstrated, conventional farming practices decrease the phenolic content.[19] A 2001 scientific review by A. Worthington of forty-one studies comparing the nutritional value of organic and conventional produce revealed that organic produce had on average 27 percent more vitamin C, 21.1 percent more iron, 29.3 percent more magnesium and 13.6 percent more phosphorous than conventional produce.[20] My patients routinely say that organic foods, whether fruit, cheese, or meat, just taste better.

If you are still unconvinced, consider the conclusions of one study that tested thirty-nine common food additives including the sweeteners saccharin and sucralose, food colors, and preservatives like BHT. The study determined that all of these substances caused DNA damage in the intestines.[21]

THE EFFECTS OF MOLD

Another common environmental hazard that affects the AS population is mold. This is directly linked to the fungal overgrowth discussed in Chapter 6. People with AS often seem to have candida or fungal overgrowth. Perhaps the worst combination is when the person has a sweet tooth, is prone to allergies, and lives in a damp area. If you are wondering if mold might be a problem, think about anxiety, irritability, or meltdown in children on rainy days or wet moldy times of the year such as in the fall. Doris Rapp suggests that the cold and flu season that seems to start each school year isn't just about children being confined in a small space with other children, but possibly also related to children being affected by the height of the mold spore stage in many parts of the country. Mold and candida are just two different types of fungi. If they build up in the body, they can disrupt the healthy intestinal balance between fungi and friendly bacteria. This may cause mental and emotional repercussions. The scientific community has explored the correlation between fungi and mental health for many years.[22] Look for mold in bathrooms, window sills in the fall, basements, and schools. In AS children, mold-related symptoms might be writing backward, anxiety, excessive silliness, or conversely, fatigue, depression, and multiple meltdowns. In AS adults, anxiety, depression, overreactivity, and volatile moods along with a whole host of physical problems, especially chronic sinus infection, athletes foot, and recurring yeast infections, are more typical.

HEAVY METALS

Along with the insecticide and pesticide chemical compounds in our foods, and mold in our bathrooms and basements, there is a corresponding awareness of the possible effects of heavy metals such as aluminum, mercury, cadmium, copper, and lead can have on mental and emotional function especially in the autism spectrum community. Researchers at the Pfeiffer Treatment Center, a prominent facility for the research and treatment of biochemical conditions, suggest that autism spectrum conditions may hinge on the body's inability to manage heavy metals both beneficial and toxic in the body.[23]

Mercury

Mercury tops the list of heavy metals that affects people with AS. While mercury is present in our environment from multiple sources including coal-burning power plants, hazardous waste disposal, and fish, most people think of vaccinations. The connection between vaccinations and conditions on the autism spectrum is a very controversial and complicated subject. There are two major concerns with vaccinations: the effects of thimerosal, a mercury-derived preservative, and the reaction in some children from the measles antibody found in measles vaccination.

Thimerosal was introduced as a vaccine preservative in the mid- to late-1930s. Several years later, in 1944, Hans Asperger first identified the syndrome in children. Once metabolized in the body, thimerosal produces ethyl mercury. Ethyl mercury was banned in the United States as a fungicide in the 1970s because of its toxicity in causing cancer, adversely affecting reproduction and development of the fetus, and its neurotoxicity. Even with this awareness, the pharmaceutical companies continued to use thimerosal in vaccinations for decades. The majority of the scientific community, the CDC (Center for Disease Control) and the IOM (Institute of Medicine), an independent research facility, attest that there is no conclusive scientific proof that vaccinations can lead to autism or AS. Even this did not soothe the concerns of parents of autistic spectrum children as the CDC commissioned the IOM study and possibly influenced its outcome. The IOM presented three reports all confirming the safety of vaccinations. Only mass pressure from the parents of autistic children has forced the removal of thimerosal from children's vaccinations. Actually, it wasn't removed, but reduced to 0.005 percent in children's vaccinations and remains in vaccinations not specifically designated as children's vaccines such as flu and tetanus at 0.01 percent level.

The pharmaceutical, government, and medical consensus was that the thimerosal would not adversely affect adults. And while this may or may not be true for the general public, in neurodevelopmental conditions such as AS, a neurotoxin such as thimerosal should be suspect. If a substance harms the nervous system, it makes sense to study these effects carefully before exposing a person with a known neurological condition such as AS to the substance.

But perhaps the reason there lacks irrefutable scientific evidence is that it would be virtually impossible to do a double blind on several thousand children, vaccinating half and not the other and then watching to see what percentage developed autistic-like behaviors. Clearly, vaccinations don't seem to adversely affect the majority of children who get them. What makes one small group of children susceptible and the larger group not? Perhaps the affected group has a genetic or familial tendency toward neurological conditions such as AS. These arguments, however, don't bring much comfort to moms like Mindy or Karen.

Mindy, an extremely gentle and kind person, married late and had her son, Michael, at forty-two years of age. At first, Michael was everything she had ever hoped for. Like his mom, he was gentle yet playful. By eighteen months, he was talking, walking, and leading what seemed a very normal happy childhood. After his eighteenth month series of vaccinations, his childhood became a nightmare. For the first two days after the vaccination, he had a 102 fever that didn't respond to medicine. During the fever, he would throw his head back and slam it into the floor. When the fever abated, Michael had completely changed in personality. He was violent, discontent, and mean to other children. By age five, he was increasingly withdrawn and avoided eye contact. He was tentatively diagnosed with Asperger Syndrome and was offered a drug regime. His mom explained that he didn't start out this way and how the vaccination seemed to change him, but doctor after doctor and behavioral therapist after therapist seemed to think this was irrelevant. Despite the lack of scientific support, Mindy is convinced that for Michael, the vaccination strongly and adversely affected his nervous system.

Sally, a very inquisitive two-year-old was her mom's (Linda) third child. Sally spoke well and had played well with other children. The only health problem Sally had was her teeth. Sally's teeth were discolored and decayed from the bottles of watered-down apple juice. The dentist took one look at Sally's mouth and said, "Thirty minutes under anesthesia or three hours in the dental chair." Wanting to spare her child the trauma, Linda elected for the anesthesia. And true to his word, the dentist had Sally in and out of the minor surgery in less than thirty minutes with twelve new mercury fillings. Within days of the surgery, Linda realized something was wrong. Sally seemed dull and anxious. She would look blank a lot and her eyes no longer sparkled with intelligence. The dentist thought Linda was imagining things; but Sally's new behavior persisted. She couldn't seem to grasp simple concepts and seemed to have unlearned earlier knowledge. Before the surgery, she could sit through and pay attention to three or four picture books; now even one book taxed her ability to stay focused. When time for kindergarten came, it was clear she was not able to keep up with the other children. As Sally's baby teeth fell out, so did the mercury fillings. But the damage wasn't rectified that easily. The mercury was now lodged in her tissue and much more difficult to remove. Sally was diagnosed at age ten with Asperger Syndrome. It took several years of homeopathy, diet, natural chelation, and a supportive family to reverse the worst effects.

The question parents like Mindy and Linda ask is what is the critical number of anecdotal reports at which point the medical community accepts the potential for serious damage in some children from thimerosal. At what point can thimerosal be taken out of all vaccinations? According to Johns Hopkins Institute for Vaccine Safety as of March 2006, thimerosal is still present in general vaccinations such as tetanus, influenza, and Diphtheria-tetanus-acellular pertussis vaccine shots.[24]

In July 2005, the U.S. Department of Health and Human Services Centers for Disease Control and Prevention presented a detailed analysis of the effects of mercury in their Third National Report on Human Exposure to Environmental Chemicals. After a thorough review of mercury toxic effect on the body, they concluded that, "finding a measurable amount of mercury in blood or urine does not mean that the level of mercury causes an adverse health effect."[25] As of 2006, mercury is still present in many common items. It is available as thimerosal in adult vaccinations such as influenza and hepatitis shots, some topical antiseptics, fish and shell-fish, dental amalgams, and some imported cosmetic skin creams. According to David Kirby in his book on the mercury debate, *Evidence of Harm*, people are also exposed to mercury via pesticides, PCBs, flame retardant fabrics, jet fuel, live viruses in vaccines, and cell phone use.[26] In the Appendix is a list of names of mercury derivatives to help you better identify it in your household items.

A question that is frequently asked by my patients is how much fish can they eat safely despite its mercury content? The best answer is to only buy fish that is routinely tested for mercury. But if you need more motivation, consider the following 2003 study by Carta in *Neurotoxicology*. The study concluded that when testing the neurological changes in two groups of people, one eating tuna and the other not, there was decreased reaction time and increased hand tremors in the tuna eaters.[27] A second study by Sanfeliu revealed even a small amount of mercury obtained by a few meals of fish per week could adversely affect neurotransmitters and trigger excitotoxins, or substances that overexcite nerve cells, in the brain.[28] In the AS person, this would result in an increase in anxiety, agitation, and overreactivity. A University of North Dakota study by Raymond et al. offers a solution.[29] Most forms of mercury, including methylmercury found in seafood bind with selenium. Selenium is a mineral that is necessary for liver detoxification to take place. Adequate intake of selenium can bind or chelate the mercury and deactivate its ability to adversely affect the nervous system. One food, the Brazilian nut, contains 780 percent of the daily recommended value of selenium. So, this food should be considered a medicine that will help remove excess mercury, but consumed in moderate amounts such as quarter cup daily for an adult as no specific guidelines have been established. In the very rare cases of selenium toxicity or selenosis, symptoms include gastrointestinal upset, hair loss, white blotchy nails, garlic breath odor, fatigue, irritability, and mild nerve damage. But mercury is not the only heavy metal to affect the nervous system.

Aluminum

For several decades, scientists have been studying the effects of aluminum in the body. And while its effects on specific conditions remain a heated debate, there are some accepted facts about aluminum. Characteristics of aluminum toxicity are stuttering, gait disturbance, myoclonic or muscle twitching jerks, seizures, coma, and abnormal EEG. There is also some speculation that aluminum interferes with calcium absorption. When this happens, calcium is excreted instead of being utilized in the bones and teeth. Aluminum can lead to an increase in copper absorption. Copper in any but trace amounts can result in yet another set of toxic symptoms including headaches, fatigue, insomnia, depression, disorientation, and learning disorders.

Aluminum accumulation can decrease levels of dopamine, norepinephrine, and 5-hydroxytryptamine, three neurotransmitters needed for stable mood and motivation, as well as contribute to memory loss, in-coordination, and mental confusion. We know that it crosses the blood-brain barrier and accumulates in the brain, as well as the lungs, liver, and kidneys. Despite thirty years of scientific research showing its adverse effects on the human nervous system, aluminum can commonly be found in aluminum cookware, beer, and soft drink cans, aluminum foil, antiperspirants, some antacids, especially if consuming citrus at the same time, buffered aspirin, in processed cheese, in the bleached flour of store-bought baked goods, as a drying agent in baking powder, in cosmetics, in some multivitamins and in our water supply as an agent to remove dirt. It is also a relatively common emission in industrial areas and a critical part of the fuel system in Space Programs' booster rockets.

Lead

Lead toxicity contributes to delayed mental development, hyperactivity, learning and attention problems, and is another heavy metal that poses a problem for people with AS. Related physical problems are fatigue, anemia, metallic taste, weight loss, headaches, insomnia, nervousness, and impaired nervous system function. Fortunately, because of the public's awareness of this health hazard, it is becoming a diminishing risk for most people. We can still find it in tap water from old lead pipes, gasoline, lead crystal, demolition sites, old paint removal, ceramics, and any environmental exposure from battery manufacture, certain food supplements such as calcium dolomite, or vitamins, or herbs from other countries. Lead poisoning can also occur when children swallow nonfood items like paint chips, fishing sinkers, curtain weights, or even bullets. The U.S. EPA warned as recently as February 2006 that even "Legally 'lead-free' plumbing may contain up to 8 percent lead. The most common problem is with brass or chrome-plated brass faucets and fixtures which can leach significant amounts of lead into the water, especially hot water."[30]

Cadmium

Cadmium is commonly found in color pigments used in plastics and paints, cigarette smoke, contaminated food, especially grains, which have absorbed the cadmium from water, soil, and fertilizers, air, and contaminated water from heavy industrial incinerators. AS-related symptoms of chronic cadmium exposure could include learning disorders, migraines, and loss of taste and smell. Other general physical symptoms are hair loss, anemia, arthritis, migraine, growth impairment, emphysema, osteoporosis, poor appetite, and cardiovascular disease.

Copper

Many people on the autism spectrum tend to have higher copper levels than the general population. A possible explanation is that they have less ceruloplasmin, a protein that binds with excess copper and aids in its excretion from the body. Excessive copper can cause high blood pressure, irritability, fatigue, hyperactivity, regular unexplained nausea, poor concentration, short-term memory lapses, joint pain and swelling, and difficulty in falling asleep. Copper maintains an inverse balance with zinc. High copper levels often suggest low zinc levels. This imbalance is common in people on the autism spectrum, which is why zinc is often supplemented in this group.

TESTING FOR HEAVY METALS AND CHEMICAL TOXINS

After reading all the overlapping symptoms of the various heavy metal toxicities, it's hard to figure out where to start. The best place to start is with the person's current exposure and history of exposure. The Environmental Protection Agency offers a link, http://www.epa.gov/epahome/commsearch.htm, which allows you to search your community by zip code for environmental toxins. This tells you what you are exposed to on a daily basis. Your exposure history presents a more complete picture. Often, the person suspects that he or she may be been exposed to heavy metals or chemicals. In one AS child's case, when his mom was pregnant with him, she was a dental assistant and around materials for amalgam fillings. In another case the person was raised in a semiindustrial area where heavy metals and chemicals were routinely released into the atmosphere by factories and plants. Sometimes, the person's symptoms seem to correspond with those of a particular or multiple chemicals. In conditions such as AS, it's easy to spend thousands of dollars testing for various substances. I tend to work with the diet, lifestyle, and immediate environment, and generally only do testing when indicated. For example, if a person eats an organic whole foods diet, exercises regularly, and takes a well-balanced regimen of vitamin and herbal supplements, has a toxin-free immediate environment and still has strong AS symptoms, there may be heavy metal or chemical toxicity. This is when it is important to test for the potential imbalance before initiating a particular detoxification treatment. All treatments except for dietary treatments can cause secondary problems if they aren't needed. For example, copper is commonly low in people on the autism spectrum and taking zinc supplements seems like an easy solution. However, if there isn't a lab confirmation of the low copper and high levels of zinc, the person may end up with anemia from excessive zinc causing excretion of iron along with the copper resulting in dizziness, inability to concentrate, nausea, and fatigue. Similarly, DMSA (dimercaptosuccinic acid) a heavy metal chelator, which is easily available over the Internet, is extremely harsh on the kidneys. It should never be used without a physician's supervision. There are several basic ways to test for heavy metals: hair, urine, and blood analyses. Your physician will help you determine which test best fits your particular situation.

Hair Analysis

Testing hair for heavy metals is the least expensive way to determine heavy metal levels over a long period of time. The EPA considers hair analysis a viable way to measure and monitor long-term heavy metal toxicity. The main concern of accuracy with hair analysis is that even if the recommended precautions of avoiding most hair-care products are followed, false positives because of daily environmental exposure to heavy metals such as off-gassing from office machinery, flooring, and furniture, among other things, may still occur. Also, if the sample isn't taken from multiple sites, it will skew the results. Finally, lab results are only as good as the lab. I have put names of some reputable labs in the Appendix.

Urine Analysis

Testing urine is another way to check for heavy metal toxicity. If you suspect that you have been exposed to heavy metals within the last few weeks, the toxins are still probably being excreted and a simple urinalysis is adequate to see how much you were affected. If the toxicity is over several months to years, then a provocative urine test is a better option. In provocative testing, a chelator, a substance that draws heavy metals out of the body such as DMSA, is administered for one to two days. This way the heavy metals are drawn out of the tissues where it is hard to measure and released into the urine. Then a urine sample is taken and sent off to a lab. The provocative test more accurately reflects the heavy metal toxicity. In the 2005 Consensus Position Paper by the Autism Research Institute (ARI), they contend that the provoked urine and stool samples are the most reliable methods.[31] The ARI additionally recommends an unprovoked urine sample should be taken first, then followed by the provoked. This would provide a personal comparison, which may be more indicative of heavy metal toxicity than simply a comparison of the person's results with the lab's baseline. The only caution with the provoked urine test is that the chelator can be a toxic substance itself. Alternatively, I've seen good results using herbal chelators. As with the hair analysis, DMSA is routinely used as a chelator, though a few doctors prefer DMPS (Dimercapto-1-sulphonate).

Stool Analysis

Just as it sounds, there are labs that use stool samples to determine levels of heavy metals and chemicals. Similar to the urine tests, a chelator as a provative agent is needed. Two prominent European dentists, Graeme Hall and Lilian Winkvist, who advocate for reduced metals in dentistry, state, "Faeces or stool are the only way of estimating metal load as the metal are bound up in the bile salts to be excreted."[32] It's a painless noninvasive test that, while somewhat messy, can be done conveniently in the home.

Blood Analysis

The body clears toxic elements from the blood fairly rapidly. It will excrete the toxins or move them to the tissues for storage. Therefore, a simple whole blood test will generally only reflect heavy metal or chemical exposure within hours, to days, to a couple of weeks. It's not a good test for long-term heavy metal or chemical toxicity.

There are several different forms of blood tests. Some labs do a straight blood test analyzing levels of the heavy metals or chemicals. Others test blood serum, or blood without cells or other particulates, for the body's immune reaction to heavy metals by determining levels of antibodies to the various substances. However, some scientists dispute the accuracy of the heavy metal tests, especially mercury. This has spawned a new form of testing called metallothionein protein screening, which has become increasingly popular within the autism population. Metallothionein is a protein that binds to heavy metals such as copper and mercury to render them harmless and hasten their excretion from the body. One theory is that in the autism populations including Asperger, metallothionein is not functioning correctly. The test checks for metallothionein levels, which reflect how well the toxins are being secreted.

The same method works when checking for chemicals. There are assorted blood serum tests looking for antibodies to chemicals such as benzene, formaldehyde (FMA), toluene di-isocyanate, and trimellitic anhydride.

Chelating Agents

Once specific heavy metals and chemicals have been identified through lab testing, the next step is to remove them. Chelation is most commonly done by pill, injection, or IV (intravenous) therapy. If taken in pill form, the chelators' effectiveness hinges on how much is being absorbed. Absorption depends on the health of the person's intestines. As we discussed earlier, the intestines are rarely functioning well in conditions such as AS that are on the autism spectrum. Another major concern with chelation is that these substances dislodge the toxins from tissue, but if the person's excretory system isn't working well, the toxins may simply move to a new location.

Standard Chelators

In the typical chelating scenario, one of several chelating agents such as DMSA or DMPS, is administered to the patient and carefully monitored. There are several reasons to monitor this process. Chelators excrete beneficial minerals such as calcium and potassium right along with the toxic ones. The doctor will both recognize signs of beneficial metals deficiency as well as know how to replenish them effectively. Second, chelating agents are not benign substances. As they remove toxins, they can cause secondary harmful effects on the kidneys.

Arguably the best-known and most readily available, DMSA has a long history of use and is particularly useful for chelating lead and mercury. It can cross the blood brain barrier and remove mercury from brain tissue. There is some debate as to whether it is safe to do DMSA chelation with mercury amalgam dental fillings. The mercury will be leached from the fillings and may lodge in the brain. Another concern is anecdotal reports of increased agitation and seizures from redistribution of mercury in the brain, especially when combined with the antioxidant alpha-lipoic acid. There are additional adverse reactions reported to DMSA, which include rash, nausea, diarrhea, anorexia, headache, dizziness, sensorimotor neuropathy, and decreased urination. Most of these seem more related to the loss of beneficial minerals rather than the DMSA itself and can be avoided with judicial replenishment of those substances. DMSA has long-standing approval by the FDA as a chelating agent. DMSA goes through the digestive system and is primarily excreted from the kidneys.

A second common chelator, DMPS, bypasses the digestive tract and is effective at chelating lead and mercury. It is gaining popularity but like all chemical chelators will remove beneficial minerals from the body. Despite its many years of use, it has not been approved by the FDA and is considered experimental. There are few reputable records on adverse effects. However, a quick survey of the Internet will show that they exist.

A chelator that has been used for fifty years, EDTA (calcium disodium ethylenediaminetetraacetate), targets heavy metals, especially lead. Like DMSA, it is excreted through the kidneys, so kidney function as well as liver function should be monitored. All three of these chelators should be treated cautiously and respected for the potentially harmful substances that they are. They should also never be taken without a physician's supervision. A final caution is that these chelators take out needed beneficial heavy metals such as calcium, magnesium, potassium, and zinc and can therefore lead to increased dysfunction in multiple systems including the digestive and nervous systems and cause symptoms such as skin lesions, which then must be addressed. Two panic-stricken parents brought their seven-year-old boy to my office after having received on-going chelation from another physician. The child had painful and itchy quarter-size lesions all over his body. These lesions were indicative of a too-rapid release of toxins. This was especially alarming as it meant the kidneys and liver were having difficulty in processing the toxins so they were forced out by the body's other excretory organ, the skin. In this case, it was important not only to temporarily stop the chelation, but also to support the kidneys and liver. Because of my concern for the long- and short-term health of the kidneys and liver, I rarely suggest these forms of chelation unless in conjunction with kidney support, replenishing the needed heavy metals such as calcium, magnesium, zinc, and potassium and adding various antioxidants. I am not convinced that starting with aggressive chelating agents such as DMSA, DMPS, and EDTA is a safe trade-off for potential future problems. Instead, I find that a diverse organic whole foods diet, along with more natural chelators, is as effective and considerably less expensive. In the few cases where these are not effective, then the potentially toxic ones can be employed.

Natural Chelators

In addition to these three, there are multiple gentler substances that are currently being used to chelate heavy metals and chemicals. These safer chelating agents include S-adenosylmethionine (SAMe), alpha-lipoic acid, glutathione, selenium, zinc, N-acetylcysteine (NAC), methionine, cysteine, alpha-tocopherol, TTFD, a synthetic derivative of thiamine or vitamin B1, and ascorbic acid. While most of these substances, have had multiple published studies showing effectiveness as chelators, none of them have adequate research to conclusively state specific claims.[33–36]

Each has its own specific attributes and cautions. For example, injectable methyl B-12 increases liver detoxification, but needs to be regularly re-dosed. Glutathione is not absorbed particularly well as a pill, but seems to work fine as a topical cream. I witnessed this firsthand at a seminar. A colleague with AS inadvertently ate some sugar in his main course and proceeded to become agitated, anxious, and experienced some vision disorientation. For him, sugar acted as a toxic chemical leading to these symptoms. There were some topical glutathione samples distributed at the seminar. A half-teaspoon dose reversed these symptoms within five to ten minutes. It was very interesting to watch this transformation.

Alpha-lipoic acid is an antioxidant that helps with heavy metal chelation but seems to worsen intestinal candida. Again, these supplements should be monitored by a physician as one or more may be inappropriate in that particular person. They should never be taken together unsupervised as the combined effect may be problematic for the patient.

Intriguing but less well-studied are the effects of whole foods and herbs on chelating heavy metals. If we review the supplements that aid in chelation, glutathione, zinc, magnesium, B complex, vitamin C, selenium, taurine, and CoQ10 (co-enzyme Q10), we can see that these are all present in an organic whole foods diet. I used to think that even a healthy diet would have very little impact on getting rid of healthy metals. I am now beginning to change my mind due to some very persistent parents of some patients of mine who taught me otherwise. Occasionally, parents will have their child tested for heavy metals but will be reluctant to have their child take the chelating agents. They often elect to serve their child an organic whole foods diet and get retested after three months. Though it has been a handful of cases so far, the children's lab tests have shown decreased levels of toxicity in all cases. In one particularly toxic case, all traces of heavy metals disappeared within a couple of years.

There has also been some research on the chelating properties of various herbs and chlorophyll. An Australian researcher, Kerry Bone et al. tested forty herbs in vitro to determine their binding capacity with the heavy metals, cadmium, lead, and mercury.[37]

Three herbs, garlic, hawthorne, and milk thistle showed high binding activity individually to these heavy metals. This activity was further increased by combining the three herbs. Earlier research of garlic and milk thistle as chelating agents further supported Bone's results. However, what was new about this research was the additive effect of combining these herbs.

Chlorella, or fresh water green algae, is another substance reputed to have chelating properties. And while there haven't been enough stringent tests to make a conclusive determination, there is some clinical and early research to show it is worth investigating further.[38–40] Dr. Joyce Young, a naturopathic physician and an authority on environmental medicine, has devised a natural chlorophyll-rich chelating nutritional system that consists of eating regular amounts of fresh organic pesto. The pesto includes parsley, basil, oregano, rosemary, cilantro, chives, and garlic. She recommends varying the ingredients to fit the meal. But these herbs aren't just rich in chlorophyll, but full of antioxidants, trace minerals, and concentrated nutrients. Parsley demonstrates a consistent ability to protect the liver.[41]

There are also miscellaneous claims attributed to various other foods including the spice turmeric. S. Daniels, a South African researcher, reported evidence in a 2004 article in the *Journal of Inorganic Chemistry* that curcumin, a substance contained in turmeric (*Curcuma longa*), was able to reduce both lead and cadmium.[42] An organic whole foods diet along with herbs and other natural substances will effectively help in detoxifying people with chemical or heavy metal toxicity.

TOXINS IN OUR WATER

Just as there are contaminants in our food, there are contaminants in our water. The only problem is that we aren't sure exactly what they are. This was summed up by the EPA in their 2003 Drinking Water program Multi-Year Plan where they stated, "The existence of many thousands of unregulated chemicals and microbes that may contaminate water at the source highlights the need to focus scientific efforts on those that may pose the greatest public health risk."[43] The best way to successfully avoid these contaminants is to avoid drinking unfiltered water. There are multiple types of home water filtration systems. The key to choosing a system is to determine if it will remove all heavy metals, bacteria, viruses, insecticides, pesticides, industrial chemicals, and solvents.

Drinking good quality water benefits you more than just avoiding another source of harmful substances. When drunk in quantities of eight to twelve cups daily, water also detoxifies the body. Water as a detoxifier doesn't include water-based beverages such as coffee, tea, or flavored waters. It means plain filtered water.

AIR POLLUTANTS

The third major source of toxins along with the contaminants in our water and food is in the air we breathe. These may include home and car air fresheners, and off-gassing from furniture, carpets, new clothing, and office equipment. Again, the impaired liver function of most people with AS, makes this a more significant problem. For example, an ordinary product like a home or car air freshener may be contributing to AS symptoms.

Most people don't associate air fresheners with impaired mental function, but they should. One of the main ingredients in air fresheners is xylene. Repeated exposure to xylene can result in balance problems, memory loss, and confusion.[44] Other common air freshener ingredients are ethanol, formaldehyde, fragrances, naphthalene, and phenol. Formaldehyde is present in virtually all aspects of building including wallboards, particle boards, paints, construction glues, and carpets. It can be detected for years after the original installation of the carpets and buildings. It's especially prevalent in motor homes and mobile homes, as many of the pre-installed furniture is made from particle board. You can also commonly find it in lipstick, toothpaste, soft drinks, shampoo, and kitchen cabinets. Formaldehyde toxicity will increase the anxiety and worsen the sleep issues in the AS population.[45] If you are wondering if you are being affected by formaldehyde, you may want to look for the concurrent physical symptoms of headaches, fatigue, runny nose, nausea, and respiratory distress. They may help serve as an indicator that the air you breathe may be affecting your mood as well. The other ingredients are similarly toxic, but my purpose here is not to target one product, but to get you to consider more than just the obvious toxins in the air. When considering the sheer extent of environmental toxicity, it can seem overwhelming. And while we may not be able to effect an immediate or direct change on the volume of toxins in our workplace or schools, we can change what is present in our homes with plants, air filters, and by simply opening windows.

DETOXING THE AIR WITH PLANTS

There are several plants that help detoxify our air. In the late 1990s, Dr. Wolverton, a former NASA scientist, conducted a two-year study on plants as natural air purifiers. He concluded that some ordinary plants were extremely effective in cleaning the air. Several other scientists have reported similar results.[46, 47] For example, spider plants and philodendrons remove formaldehyde from the air; while English Ivy and Chrysanthemums minimize the effects of benzene from new plastics. Dwarf date palms removed xylene from the air. When I moved into my current office, I was concerned about the effects of toxins from the renovations on my patients and myself. I hung several plants in each room and was pleasantly surprised how effective they were. And while this may work in homes and small business offices, air filtration systems are better for more conventional settings. One of my patients became increasingly anxious over the week or so returning to work after the offices had been renovated. His company frowned on plants and he worked in a cubicle and wasn't sure how the air quality could be affected. We decided to try herbs to help detoxify his liver and an air filtration unit, which we placed right next to him in the cubicle, and directed it at him. It worked well and his symptoms decreased noticeably. Some PTA (parent, teacher associations) purchase air filters for the classrooms, especially in winter when the windows are closed.

One topic that frequently arises with the issue of air pollution is office politics. I recommend that the employee not mention AS and simply say that they are getting recurrent headaches or whatever the physical symptoms accompanying the increased anxiety are, and that he would like a trial period to see if he could be more productive with these items. If you have a long daily commute and are wondering whether the air in your car is affecting you, you might want to consider car air filters. Finally, there are environmental specialists who can determine whether air pollution is a problem in your particular area as well as HVAC (heating, ventilating, and air conditioning) consultants. The U.S. EPA will tell you exactly what the local air pollutants are for your zip code on their Web site.

FLUORESCENT LIGHTING

Fluorescent lights abound in our schools and office workplaces. For some people, fluorescent lights can adversely affect the sleep cycle, cause headaches, incite hyperactive behavior, decrease the ability to concentrate, or just make the person feel irritable and uneasy. This isn't new information. Dr. Fritz Hollwich, a German researcher first advocated a decreased use of fluorescent lights because his studies in the early 1970s showed an increase in ACTH (a cortisol-related stress hormone) levels from prolonged exposure.[48] His work pioneered many other researchers resulting in Germany instituting a ban on cool-white fluorescent lights in their hospitals and workplaces. More specific to AS, as early as 1976, scientists such as R. S. Coleman, F. Frankel, E. Ritvo, and B. J. Freeman studied the effects of fluorescent versus incandescent lights on the autism population.[49] They concluded that fluorescent lights intensified some autistic behavioral traits including repetitive behavior by increased arousal. A more recent study also demonstrates the effect of fluorescent lights on the autism spectrum population.[50] This becomes more understandable when we consider that fluorescent lights require a high-voltage discharge to be produced within the tube. They also produce magnetic fields that are significantly higher than incandescent light bulbs. In his book, *Cross Currents*, Robert Becker, MD, wrote, "The 10-watt fluorescent lamp produces a magnetic field at least twenty times greater than a 60-watt incandescent bulb."[51] John Ott was writing medical journal articles even in the 1970s that questioned the influence of fluorescent lights on hyperactivity and learning disabilities.[52] However, research suggests that people are not uniformly affected by fluorescent lights, but when they are, it can be significant.

Patty, a forty-three-year-old research scientist with AS visited a friendly colleague's office for the first time. She was excited about the visit, as she was interested in the new information her colleague had to show her. But after about one hour, Patty noticed that she was getting tired and jumpy. She was having trouble following what was being said. Fortunately, she was able to assess the situation and determined that it was the fluorescent lights. Turning the fluorescent lights off, she felt less anxious immediately and completely regained her equilibrium within a few minutes.

I noticed this same effect while talking with a group of Asperger adults. As soon as the fluorescent lights were turned off, there was a visible relaxation in the room and increased participation in the conversation. One solution is for schools and workplaces to install full spectrum fluorescent tubes. However, this can be expensive. Some offices allow small lamps or have a lamp built into the cubicle that could be replaced with a full spectrum or even an incandescent light.

Fluorescent lights, along with computers, microwaves, high-power electric wires, and even thunderstorms are examples of EMF or electromagnetic fields. The effect of electro-magnetic fields on human health has long been debated. Both sides are fierce in the convictions and there are many excellent books written on this subject. In my practice, I find that in the AS population, most are affected by EMFs, mainly because of their heightened sensory sensitivity. I often suggest that they do a simple test. Sit and read under a fluorescent light most often found in the kitchen, and do the same thing with the fluorescent light turned off and an incandescent or a full spectrum light turned on. If you don't notice a difference than this might not be an area that affects you.

WHAT ELSE?

Look around your house and office for less obvious forms of environmental substances that may be exacerbating you or your child's symptoms. For example, play dough, face painting, and most Easter egg dyes all contain chemical toxins. The skin is not a protective barrier against these substances. Fortunately, there are safe equivalents to them all that are available either online or at your local health food store.

Maintaining a weed-free lawn may be hazardous to your health. Paraquat and rotenone, two common ingredients in lawn care, can cause confusion, muscle tremors, incoordination, and stupor. An important point to remember is that AS is a condition of the nervous system. These substances target the nervous system, and people with AS have to be additionally careful around them.

TIPS TO MINIMIZE HEAVY METAL EXPOSURE

1. Avoid sources of heavy metals such as aluminum cookware, antiperspirants, beer and soft drink cans, aluminum foil, some antacids especially if consumed with citrus, buffered aspirin, in processed cheese, in bleached flour, as a drying agent in baking powder, and some cosmetics.
2. Don't drink water from the tap. Get a water purification system. Even a simple charcoal filtration system will help.
3. Eat a varied and organic whole foods diet.
4. Avoid Dolomite, a common calcium supplement, which often contains significant amounts of arsenic, mercury, lead, and cadmium.
5. Avoid unnecessary vaccinations. Consider carefully the risk versus benefit of getting a flu shot, which as of 2006 still contains thimerosol.
6. Buy houseplants such as spider plants to protect against formaldehyde, and English Ivy against benzene.
7. Use full spectrum lights whenever possible.
8. Use a low-toxin equivalent for all your painting and remodeling needs.

It initially seems overwhelming to consider the environmental toxicity. But if you tackle it one area at a time, it becomes less daunting. We may not be able to control what is allowed in the general environment, but to some degree, we can control what we eat, breathe, drink, and keep in our own homes.

CHAPTER 9

Deer in the Headlights–Dealing with Anxiety, Depression, and Sleep

In Asperger Syndrome (AS), the nervous system is ramped up a little too much. Think about a car in idle. There are low idles and high idles—and then there are Asperger idles. The Asperger idle is extremely high and if he takes the foot off the brake, he may overreact, have an anxiety attack, or if he's a child, have a meltdown. Unfortunately, most AS people, especially children, have trouble holding their foot on the brake. Their oversensitive nervous system often has poor controls manifesting in a multitude of different nervous behaviors.

In addition to often having poor control over anxiety, the person with AS will have numerous other symptoms related to the nervous system. Think about a physical condition such as arthritis. Arthritis may have symptoms ranging from swelling, difficulty moving a joint, stiffness, and burning, aching, or sharp pain. The person with AS may often have extreme anxiety along with nervous mannerisms, sleep issues, and a high incident of depression. Fortunately, there are many ways in which natural medicine can calm the nervous system, modulate all these symptoms, and keep that foot firmly on the brake until it's time for the car to move forward smoothly.

ANXIETY

One of the most challenging aspects of AS anxiety. In fact, the average person with AS will list it as their worst complaint. One computer consultant said, "I can live with being odd, dressing unfashionably and not fitting in, but I hate the anxiety that seems to follow me wherever I go." The anxiety can be extremely debilitating. Some will hide in their cubicles at work or in the libraries at school, while others will avoid any and all social interactions. A young man, very excited to join his teammates at a victory dinner, circled the block of the restaurant six times before driving back home. His fear of saying or doing something wrong and embarrassing himself was overwhelming.

Even with friends and family, people with AS will suddenly run out of things to say. It's as if they are having a "social freeze." Many describe it as things become surreal—as if they are watching themselves become increasingly uncomfortable. This "social freeze" can come and go and is different for each person. One might be able to easily handle ninety minutes of a family get together, while another will have had their limit after thirty minutes. It's most often not a sign that they don't like the company, but that they have reached a level of discomfort within themselves in the situation.

And if that wasn't enough, the anxiety often has a physical manifestation as well. Most commonly in my office I will see tics, stammering, patients picking at things, others, or themselves, nail biting, and all sorts of involuntary hand gestures and vocalizations. In some cases, the nervous mannerism is serious enough for the diagnosis of Tourette's Syndrome. In children, these nervous mannerisms are very obvious, in adults less so. For example, one man grew a beard in his early twenties to cover up a need to stroke his chin. A woman picked out her eyelashes, but wore false eyelashes during the day. These mannerisms tend to go through cycles, for as the person is trained out of one, they develop a new one. For example, a child might start with picking at his clothes. When repeatedly reprimanded, he might then start to stammer. Psychologists call these involuntary gestures "stims," referring to nonsexual self-stimulating behaviors, and work with the person to stop doing them. People with AS often regard the mannerisms as benign energy releases.

> When she gets cold or excited, Mary, will tense every muscle in her body, shudder, and press her hands against each other, and then to her mouth. If she was very excited, for example when watching an action movie, she would also let out a whoop. When she was little, her large family would affectionately refer to this behavior as "jiggling." Gradually, Mary learned that "jiggling" was considered a little odd by nonfamily members, so, she learned to temper this in public, but continued to use "jiggling" as a nervous release. It didn't seem to affect her life at all. Married, with four adult children and a husband of twenty-seven years, Mary is a Certified Public Accountant with AS. Neither her husband nor non-AS children thought of this behavior as anything but idiosyncratic. As Mary commented, "'Jiggling' may look and sound silly, but it has helped me cope over the years and is a lot easier on my body than drugs or alcohol."

In Mary's case, her nervous mannerism was underplayed in her childhood, and though it stayed a part of her life, she was able to keep it in control in public and it didn't impact her ability to live a full and rewarding life. Steven's case was much different.

When Steven was young, his successful parents were embarrassed by his tics. When overexcited, he would tune out and make odd hand gestures anywhere from five to twenty seconds. It became a real issue in the family. Repeatedly punished for this tic, Steven began to stutter and bed-wet instead. And though his bed-wetting resolved in a few years, his stuttering continued into his adult life. His parents certainly didn't mean to make Steven feel bad about himself, but nevertheless, the message they were giving him was that he was defective.

This is a theme I have seen repeatedly, the severity of the symptom will to a certain degree be based on how it was treated in the person's early childhood.

There is a good reason for these behaviors. While scientists are just beginning to piece together a true understanding of what changes AS causes in the brain, we do know that the AS brain, as with any neurodevelopmental condition, differs from the non-AS brain. This is most noticeable in several areas including the frontal cortex (abstract thought, planning, organizing, problem solving, selective attention, and personality), prefrontal lobe (inhibitory controls), hippocampus (memory), and parts of the limbic system (emotion and motivation), especially the amygdala (emotion regulator), parahippocampal gyrus (emotional and visceral or instinctual responses), and the cerubellum (coordination, balance, manual dexterity, and gait). Interestingly, a small 2006 study demonstrated that the parents of AS children also have atypical brain function compared to the same number of sex-matched controls, which supports a family disposition to the condition.[1]

One of the results of these changes in the brain is that people with AS tend to have an overactive nervous system because the "drive" or sympathetic nervous system is always on. Commonly referred to as the "fight or flight" system, the sympathetic nervous system prepares the person to defend or run away. This would include signs such as increased perspiration including sweaty palms, tensed muscles, accelerated heart rate, and pupil dilation for better sight. The adrenal gland receives a message from the brain and secretes adrenaline (epinephrine) and norepinephrine. At the same time, the whole digestive process slows down. The salivary glands, stomach, intestines, and pancreas decrease their secretion of substances like hydrochloric acid, enzymes, and other substances that are necessary for proper digestion. With AS, you might have a person trying to carry on a mundane conversation in the schoolyard or workplace, while adrenalin is coursing through their body telling them that they are in a life and death situation. This exaggerated response of hypervigilance seems worse in children than in adults.

If the sympathetic system is overstimulated for years, certain physical conditions may develop. Prolonged anxiety can lead to high blood pressure, coronary heart disease, and sleep disturbances. A 2005 University of Pennsylvania cohort study supports this. Comparing almost 40,000 people with panic disorder with the same number without, they determined that there is a twofold risk of getting coronary heart disease in those with panic disorders.[2] The symptoms and signs for a panic disorder are increased heart rate, chest pain or discomfort, changes in breathing, fear of going crazy or losing control, dizziness, sweating, and shaking. All these symptoms are frequently found in AS patients.

In addition to the more obvious signs of anxiety, there can be difficulty in both falling and staying asleep as well as restless limbs in children and adults. Sometimes, this is less obvious in adults, as many use sleeping pills. It's almost as if the person is unwilling or unable to turn the vigilance switch off.

DEPRESSION

In addition to anxiety, depression is fairly common in AS and usually starts in late adolescence. By this time, the teenager has realized his deficiencies in social skills, his earlier school friends have moved on, and his oddities are no longer considered "cute." Sometimes there is a change of status within his birth family. The parents grow weary of accommodating his idiosyncrasies and often want the young adult out of the house. Often the person with AS is so demoralized by repeated social and professional rejection that depression sets in. When the depression is a result of the condition, then the same treatments that help with anxiety will also help with depression.

In other cases, depression can be an independent issue from AS. Several family members, with or without AS, will have a tendency toward depression. Natural medicine can help considerably, but should be overseen by a practitioner specializing in treating mental health issues.

If the depression is unrelenting, then consider pyroluria. It is frequently found in people on the autism spectrum, with ADHD, bipolar disorders, and other mental health conditions.

RULING OUT PYROLURIA

Pyroluria, a familial or hereditary blood abnormality that occurs in about 6–10 percent of the population, develops when excessive amounts of a substance called krytopyrroles is produced in the body. Harmless in low levels, krytopyrroles in higher levels bind with B-6 and zinc, blocking their absorption in the body leading to their excretion in the urine. When this happens, symptoms such as fear, anxiety, poor stress coping skills, and overreactivity can occur. Stress exacerbates pyroluria. For example, young people leaving for college or the military, parents divorcing, or the ending of serious relationships can all trigger these symptoms. As the condition progresses, the person become increasingly depressed and withdrawn. And yet, unlike many conditions, the person with pyroluria will have a sense that something biological is wrong. Another way to tell the difference is that the person with pyroluria will also not respond to conventional antidepressants affecting serotonin levels, while the person with AS will.

Here is a quick questionnaire to help you determine if pyroluria may be present.

1. Do you tend to skip breakfast or have morning nausea?
2. Do you have or have you ever had persistent constipation?
3. Do you have white spots on your nails?
4. Did you get a "stitch" in your side when you ran as a child?
5. Do you or did you have moderate to severe acne as a teenager?
6. Do you have pain in your knees?
7. Do you have cold hands and feet?
8. Do you have stretch marks as an adolescent or adult even without a large weight gain or loss?
9. Are your teeth or were your teeth before orthodontic treatment crowded with teeth growing over teeth?
10. Did puberty start a little later for you than others?
11. Do you find that conventional antidepressants don't work for you?
12. Do you tend toward apathy?
13. Do you have a tendency toward iron-deficiency anemia or test borderline?
14. Do you have nightmares?
15. Do you have tingling sensations or even tremors in your arms or legs?
16. Do you tend to have paler skin than other family members?
17. Do you tend to get overwhelmed in stressful situations?
18. Do you feel that there must be a biological reason, rather than a situational reason, for your depression?

If you have answered "yes" to at least ten of these questions and you think the overview of pyroluria fits your situation, then there is a simple urine test to determine if you have the condition. This test can be ordered through a physician or directly by the patient. Pyroluria may exist by itself or with other neurological conditions such as AS and can be detected with a simple urine lab test that measures krytopyrroles. Information on this lab test is in the Appendix.

The treatment is straightforward, large doses of pryroxidine (B-6) and zinc along with some other trace minerals to compensate for the lost B-6 and zinc. Usually the improvement is quite dramatic and will start within seventy-two hours of supplementing the B-6 and zinc, though it may take weeks to a couple of months to completely stabilize the person. Also, B-6 works with the other B-vitamins, so it is important to take a B-complex or a multivitamin with B-vitamins in it so that a different form of B-vitamin imbalance doesn't occur.

Sometimes, the person is unable to absorb the B-6 in pill form and must take it in liquid or injection form until they heal their intestines and the absorption improves. Because this is familial, it will be lifelong, and without the B-6 and zinc, the person will revert to the anxious depressed state within two to three weeks.

Even if you think you have pyroluria and are tempted to go ahead and just start taking the B-6 and zinc at these very high doses, please don't. If pyroluria isn't present, then taking B-6 and zinc at high levels can lead to a host of problems. Prolonged high levels of zinc can lead to anemia, nausea, vomiting, fever, and an increased risk of autoimmune conditions. Excessive B-6 can result in loss of coordination of the muscles when walking, an internal vibration, light-sensitive sores, and numbness of the hands or feet.

TREATING ANXIETY AND DEPRESSION

In natural medicine, there are many ways to treat anxiety and depression including diet, amino acids, herbs, vitamins, and homeopathy. Like conventional medicine, natural medicine is used in conjunction with therapy. I share patients with several therapists and they will tell me how obvious it is when the patient isn't keeping up with the diet and treatment plan and how quickly they regain their improvement when they return to it.

The most important thing you can do to control depression is to follow the dietary recommendations in Chapter 7. Whether you are taking conventional antidepressants or natural medicine, both are more effective with a healthy diet that supports the nervous system. In addition to a healthy diet, amino acids, herbs, vitamins, minerals, essential fatty acids, and various supplements will help with the anxiety and depression. It's important to start with a good multivitamin/mineral supplement.

Most people don't know how to determine the quality of a multivitamin/mineral. There are several key indicators on the bottle that will help you. First, make sure it is in capsule form. Many people with or without AS have impaired digestion and may have insufficient stomach acids to break down a pill, but enough to release the contents of a capsule. Look at the fillers; they will be listed under "other ingredients." A good multivitamin won't contain magnesium stearate, stearic acid, or ascorbyl palmitate. These are fillers designed to help the product better flow through the machinery. Other fillers might also include coloring, aluminum derivatives, sugars such as glucose, lactose, or glucose, and even the plastic propylene glycol. Something else to consider is the form of calcium. Calcium comes in many forms with varying degrees of absorbability. Currently calcium hydroxyapetite followed by calcium citrate or aspartate appears to be the best absorbed.

These are just general guidelines as there are many factors that wouldn't be obvious from the label. As a general rule, don't buy a bargain multivitamin. And if you want to know if your vitamin at home is helping, stop taking it for three to seven days. You should notice a drop in well-being during that time.

Along with a good multivitamin, amino acids are a potent medicine to treat anxiety and depression. Amino acids exist in all forms of protein foods such as meat, nuts, beans, fish, eggs, poultry, and dairy. When taken as isolated supplements, the amino acids l-tryptophan, gamma-aminobutyric acid (GABA), dl-phenylalanine, and l-tyrosine have specific effects on the nervous system. They either act directly or convert into neurotransmitters that send different messages to parts of the brain. L-tryptophan and GABA send inhibitory messages to calm the brain, while dl-phenylalanine and l-tyrosine send signals to stimulate the brain. Establishing the correct balance is important. For example, the person with AS needs to calm the brain to decrease the anxiety, but needs to stimulate the brain to increase motivation. Long-term, amino acids need to be used cautiously and under the supervision of a physician knowledgeable in this area. This specialist will be able to test for deficiencies so that the treatment will be that much more effective. Often more than one may be needed and then in varying amounts, at different times of the day, and for different lengths of time. Some amino acids compete with each other and should be taken separately. Others can interact with herbs and should be used cautiously. All amino acids require a healthy diet or at least a good multivitamin and mineral to supply the necessary nutrients to make the amino acids work effectively. When used correctly, they can dramatically improve the person's outlook and quality of life. In general, amino acids shouldn't be taken when using conventional medication, as they will interact with each other as they are both working on the same neurotransmitters. The only exception to this is if the use of both is being overseen by a physician skilled in this area.

While serving a similar function to conventional antidepressants by increasing serotonin levels, amino acids act somewhat differently on the body. For one thing, they replenish low levels of serotonin, dopamine, or norepinephrine and are often not needed long-term. Conventional antidepressants recirculate existing serotonin supplies, some of which are then excreted out the body. Unlike conventional drugs, amino acids can be discontinued at any time without withdrawal symptoms. Conventional antidepressants must be weaned off when discontinuing to avoid serious withdrawal symptoms but have a much longer effect than simple amino acids. Amino acids have a six-hour half-life and must be taken at least twice daily for most people.

Most importantly, if used correctly, amino acids are safe in all age groups. In late 2005, the FDA requested all manufacturers of antidepressants to put a warning on their products that there may be an increased risk of suicide or suicidal thinking in children and adolescents who take their products. Amino acids are a safe and effective alternative to these drugs.

While there are many more amino acids than I will discuss here, the following is a brief explanation of four amino acids, l-tryptophan, gamma-aminobutyric acid (GABA), dl-phenylalanine, and l-tyrosine, which I have found the most helpful in treating those with AS.

L-tryptophan

Most people recognize the neurotransmitter serotonin. Serotonin is the substance the conventional antidepressants strive to increase in brain circulation as it improves the mood. L-tryptophan is a precursor of serotonin. However, l-tryptophan must first convert into 5-hydroxytryptophan (5-HTP), which then converts to serotonin.

l-tryptophan→ 5-HTP→ Serotonin

This is an important distinction. The closer a substance is to the final product, the more drug-like its effects. For example, tryptophan can go in multiple pathways other than the conversion to serotonin; 5-HTP is pretty much locked into a single conversion to serotonin. When someone takes l-tryptophan, their body decides how much will be converted to serotonin in the 5HTP rate-limiting step. With 5HTP, it will essentially all get converted into serotonin. One study showed that long-term administration of serotonin resulted in a buildup in the heart and led to heart valve disease.[3] While this is rarely problematic, it's a good idea to either use the more expensive l-tryptophan or alternate between the two forms.

L-tryptophan or 5-HTP improves mood very quickly. Both work better if taken on an empty stomach or with a simple carbohydrate such as a single saltine cracker. If taken with protein-containing food, l-tryptophan will bind with the other amino acids in the food and very little will convert to serotonin. For some, 5-HTP can cause nausea because it metabolizes in the stomach. If that happens, eat a cracker. Foods in which l-tryptophan occurs naturally are turkey, beef, dairy, chicken, eggs, wild game, nutritional yeast, bananas, sunflower, sesame and pumpkin seeds, lentils, split peas, all types of dried beans, brazil nuts, cashews, filberts, peanuts, and wheat germ—which gives you another reason to eat a varied and healthy diet. Also, slow repetitive exercises such as tai chi, yoga, or even breathing exercises increase serotonin levels.[4]

In addition to treating depression, l-tryptophan and 5-HTP are also effective in some people to calm anger outbursts, treat anxiety, obsessive-compulsive tendencies, and help with insomnia. The average adult dosage of l-tryptophan is 500–2000 mg daily, usually in divided doses. For example a person might take 1000 mg before breakfast and then another 1000 mg before bedtime. I tend to use herbs with very young children to treat these conditions, but it is common to treat teenagers with similar doses. As 5-HTP has a more potent effect, you dose it considerably lower. For example, an average 150 lb adult would take 100–200 mg a day in divided doses. I find that it helps decrease depression and insomnia very quickly. But its effect on anxiety, obsessive-compulsive tendencies, and anger outbursts take longer. Dr. Joan Mathews Larson, who runs the Health Recovery Center in Minnesota and is author of *Depression-Free Naturally*, states it can take two weeks before the person becomes noticeably calmer after starting the l-tryptophan.[5]

If you take l-tryptophan or 5-HTP on your own and it doesn't seem to help, it may be because serotonin level either isn't your problem or it isn't your only amino acid deficiency. Or another condition such as pyroluria exists concurrently with the AS. It could even be that your basic nutrition is insufficient and you are not getting enough trace minerals to make the amino acids work.

Caution Box

Never exceed the recommended dose on the bottle of the 5-HTP or l-tryptophan or combine it with SSRIs, MAO inhibitors, or any conventional medication that increases the amount of serotonin circulating in the brain without supervision by a medical practitioner trained in amino acids, as excessive serotonin can be toxic. When there is an excessive serotonin, it can be a medical emergency. Often the person may become confused and agitated. He may also have a headache, shivering, high blood pressure, rapid heartbeat, nausea, diarrhea, sweating, muscle twitching, and tremors.

Some people respond very well to l-tryptophan for about three days and then get very drowsy during the day. This indicates an imbalance in multiple neurotransmitters and is often improved by adding dl-phenylalanine or l-tyrosine.

Dl-phenylalanine

Dl-phenylalanine works best for those who are slow getting started in the morning, overly sensitive, easily disappointed, or who cry easily. The people who seem to need it most often crave dark chocolate, a natural source of this amino acid. Other sources are dairy products, cottage cheese, chicken, duck, ricotta, soybeans, turkey, walnuts, and wild game. Coffee decreases it. Dl-phenylalanine doesn't work well in hyperactive people as it may increase their symptoms. It's better for the person with AS who has a tendency toward ADD (attention deficit disorder) rather than ADHD (attention deficit *hyperactivity* disorder).

Common doses for a 150 lb person are 500 mg one to three times a day on an empty stomach. Again, I tend to use herbs in very young children, but smaller doses can be used for children ten years and over. With children, it is better to have a physician monitor the situation.

L-tyrosine

For people who don't crave chocolate or seem oversensitive but seem to need help getting up in the morning, l-tyrosine is another option. L-tyrosine is the amino acid involved with motivation. It's really effective for sluggish and easily distracted people. They tend to be burnt out and mildly or moderately depressed. Tyrosine must convert into a different substance called dopamine to accomplish that job. Tyrosine is found in the diet in meat sources as well as fish, soy products, avocados, bananas, dairy products, lima beans, and sesame seeds.

Even more than l-tryptophan, the use of tyrosine should be monitored by a physician specializing in amino acids. Tyrosine should be avoided in those with high blood pressure or who are on MAO inhibitors or antipsychotic medications. It's also better to not use tyrosine with those who have self-injurious behavior. While this behavior is often done in private by adults, in children, it may occur as head banging or pulling out hair (trichotillomania) and in some cases, can seem harmless as if the child is playing a game. I've seen a few parents shake their head with bemused expressions as their child repeatedly hits himself.

In some people, tyrosine can cause headaches. In those instances, it is better to take tyrosine in the form of acetyl-l-tyrosine to avoid headaches. It should be avoided in those with liver disease including hepatitis or cirrhosis. If tyrosine is taken in excessively high doses, it can cause nausea, vomiting, diarrhea, or extreme nervousness. The most important caution with tyrosine is if you have a personal or family history of the skin cancer, malignant melanoma. It can increase the division of these types of cancerous cells. Again, these are extremely rare and happen almost exclusively with an abuse of this amino acid. The only side effect I have ever seen in my patients is headaches, which can easily be avoided by using acetyl-l-tryrosine or dl-phenylalanine. However, I tend to use this amino acid short-term or in very low doses for longer periods. Despite all these warnings, if used correctly, l-tyrosine works effectively to help with motivation. If you fit the profile described above and tyrosine doesn't help, then it may be your adrenals or thyroid may need support and you should address this with your doctor.

GABA (gamma-aminobutyric acid)

GABA is perhaps the best amino acid for calming the brain from anxiety, tics, or even seizures. Virtually every person I have ever seen with AS benefits from a moderate supplementation of GABA. It also helps in cases where the person is tired all day, has cold extremities, and high blood pressure—results of anxiety sustained for years. I most often use it in a pill formulation, which includes herbs and vitamins as I find it works extremely well that way. Under physician supervision, it is safe for children over eight-years-old.

> Roger, a very sensitive little boy with AS, hated to go to school. Between his difficulty with reading and his desire to do well in his school assign-ments, he worked himself up into a stressful state. So much so that he was locked into a rigid way of thinking that was impervious to his parents' sug-gestions or teacher's help. Each morning, he would get an anxiety-related stomachache anticipating the day and sometimes, he even developed the stomachache the night before a school day. Along with dietary changes, we recommended taking a GABA formulation each morning and evening on an empty stomach. By the end of the week, his stomachaches were gone. He still needed to work on his reading, but he was now better to accept the help from his parents and teacher.

A very basic guideline for a 150 lb person is 200 mg three times a day on an empty stomach. GABA can be found in combination products in amounts ranging from 25 mg–200 mg.

This is a brief overview of four amino acids. There are many more. I have listed a few excellent books in the Appendix, which will help you to understand how to use them correctly. Amino acids can be deceptively easy to use and are readily available. However, they can be overused. It can take years before a practitioner becomes proficient in their use after seeing hundreds of patients; it's best to work with someone who has experience in their use.

Herbs

Herbs are another great tool in treating AS. Think of them as highly specialized proprietary medicines that contain vitamins, minerals, amino acids, and various other nutrients that help them work safely and effectively. Each has multiple effects on the body and each seems to work best in certain types of people. Unlike amino acids, which require minerals to work, the minerals are built right into the herbs so they can work with or without other supplementation. They don't have a pronounced drug-like effect and can be discontinued at any time with no withdrawal. Herbs are designed to be taken for relatively short periods such as two to three months and work best when alternated every two to three months. That means it's fine to use an herb or combination of herbs for two to three months, then take a break for a month before continuing again. This helps it work more effectively as the body tends to get used to repeated use.

Herbs are so readily available that most people don't realize that there are huge differences in quality. One anxious patient responded extremely well to kava. Forgetting her bottle when she went on her vacation, she bought some from a large discount chain and quickly found that she needed to take four pills instead of the one pill she had been taking from the brand she had started out with. Because herbs aren't regulated by the FDA, there are varying standards of quality. Some herbal supplement companies, including many of the large pharmaceuticals, buy herbs based on the amount of a single or a couple constituents. For example, the leaf and the root may both contain the same constituent, but the other constituents in the leaf may be mildly toxic, while those in the root are completely safe. Most pharmaceutical companies don't employ herbalists and aren't aware of these potentially serious distinctions. They may buy the leaf and not the root because of the price. Though I routinely use more than these few herbs, the following is a guide to the best researched herbs to treat anxiety and depression.

Kava (*Piper methysticum*)

For hundreds of years, the people of Micronesia, Polynesia, and Fuji have used kava for a multitude of conditions, including anxiety. Within a few years of its introduction into Western markets, it has shown its effectiveness both in slowing down racing and anxious thoughts as well as relaxing the body. It's used for both anxiety and insomnia.

Kava increases both GABA and serotonin levels. Under the scientific community's scrutiny, it has tested very well. In an eight-week randomized, referenced-control double blind clinical trial, 129 outpatients received 400 mg kava, 10 mg Buspirone (BuSpar) or 100 mg Opipramol, a common European drug for treating anxiety, for eight weeks. Kava was well-tolerated and as effective as Buspirone and Opipramol in treating generalized anxiety disorder.[6] In another placebo-controlled double blind outpatient trial, fifty patients who were treated with 100 mg of kava had a significant reduction in anxiety versus the placebo. There were no adverse effects during the trial or withdrawal symptoms when kava was discontinued.[7] Kava is a safe alternative to the extremely effective but addictive benzodiazepines such as Xanax, Klonopin, and Activan.

It's best to do a trial of kava to see how it will effect your particular constitution. Some people get vivid dreams for a few evenings. One woman, raised on a farm, said when she started kava, she dreamed she was back on the farm and could both touch and smell the cows!

Valerian (*Valeriana officialis*)

Like kava, valerian affects both GABA and serotonin receptors and therefore is good for both anxiety and for sleep. There are over ten different compounds within the herb that account for these effects. Valerian is an herb that people seem to love or hate. It seems to be most effective for wired, jumpy, and nervous people. In small doses valerian decreases their anxiety and in larger doses helps them fall asleep. Some people really don't seem to do well with valerian. In my experience, people who don't fit that wired and nervous description are in this group. Even though both valerian and kava both affect serotonin and GABA levels, each has a noticeably different effect on most people and often seem to work best together. When combined with kava, valerian seems to serve the AS community extremely well. Valerian is most often combined with other herbs in amounts from 25 mg–200 mg. It has a fairly offensive odor and is rarely drunk as a tea.

Lemon Balm (*Melissa Officialis*)

Lemon balm or melissa is a wonderful and gentle herb that has repeatedly shown in scientific studies its effectiveness in treating anxiety. In one double-blind, placebo-controlled study, Drs. Kennedy, Little, and Scholey, researchers from the University of Northumbria in Britain, found that lemon balm not only helped students cope with test anxiety, but it also helped them increase the speed of the mathematical calculations without a decrease in accuracy.[8] In an earlier study testing higher doses, the same researchers discovered that while 1600 mg of lemon balm provided the most anxiety-decreasing effect, the lower doses of 600 and 1000 mg improved memory performance.[9] When these researchers combined lemon balm with valerian in a 2006 study, the results were even better especially when lower amounts of each were used in combination.[10] Lemon balm is a good choice for those who might need extra help with improving their ability to focus as well as decrease their anxiety.

Sally is a thirty-year-old mother of two children. In addition to her intense shyness and anxiety, she always seemed befuddled. One day, she arrived at my office about thirty minutes before her scheduled office visit, completely distraught. We had some fresh lemon balm from the garden and we made her a cup of tea while she waited. By the time I finished with the earlier patient and was ready to see her, she was a completely different person. She smiled and said, "What did you put into that tea?"

And while not everyone is going to respond that quickly or that well, lemon balm is a very useful herb in the treatment of anxiety, especially if present with mental confusion.

Like all herbs, lemon balm has multiple effects on the body. For example, in addition to being an anxiolytic and sleeping medicine, it has antiviral, antioxidant cholesterol-lowering effects as well as the ability to increase glutathione, a nutrient needed for detoxification. It also helps improve digestion by decreasing the tendency toward gas. And it's safe enough to be used in very young children. Further, lemon balm protects the liver. This is an important consideration when the person is taking conventional drugs or ingesting any other substance that will provide extra stress to the liver.

A common dose for a 150 lb person is 600–800 mg; for a 75 lb child 300–400 mg daily. A higher dose will increase the sense of calm but will add a sedative effect. This may be desirable at night. As its name suggests, lemon balm has a mild lemony taste, so the leaves can be given in tea form to young children. The plant is readily available and grows well in most temperate climates. The leaves are the part of the plant with the most anxiolytic properties and can be taken in tea, tincture, or pill form. A tea made of three to six tea leaves will soothe a stressed child or adult. In lower doses, it will decrease anxiety, in higher doses it will help with insomnia.

Persons who benefit most from the use of lemon balm are shy, very anxious and insecure, slightly withdrawn persons, who tend to blame themselves rather than others.

Passionflower (*Passiflora incarnata*)

While lemon balm is best for the withdrawn AS person, passionflower is much more suited for the adult or child who tends to dramatically overreact to rather than withdraw from stress. In a 2001 randomized double blind study, passionflower compared favorably to oxazepam, an effective but habit-forming anxiety medication.[11] Passionflower took longer than oxazepam to achieve the reduction in anxiety, but it affected the job performance less. Unlike kava or lemon balm, in most cases, passionflower will not have an immediate effect, but works extremely well after it builds up over a week or two. With *Passiflora*, the flowers, leaves, and stems all help decrease anxiety, while the roots have no effect.

Passionflower is also useful for anxiety-related insomnia because of its antispasmodic and sedative qualities. Traditionally, passionflower is more effective in maintaining sleep rather than helping the person fall asleep. This was confirmed in a 1988 animal study in which passionflower prolonged the duration of sleep. Passionflower is often combined with kava or valerian.

In addition to its benefit in treating anxiety and anxiety-related insomnia, passionflower has shown in multiple studies to be effective in decreasing the withdrawal effects of various drug-addictions including benzodiazepines, nicotine, alcohol, and caffeine. In several cases, not only did the passionflower diminish the withdrawal symptoms but also maintained the same level of anxiety-decreasing activity as the drug being withdrawn.

Bacopa (*Bacopa monniera*)

An herb native to India, bacopa has been used for hundreds of years for depression, anxiety, epilepsy, and improved mental function. In several scientific studies, bacopa relaxed the body, and improved mental function without hindering coordination. It appears to help with short-term memory more than long-term. When tested with phenytoin, an epileptic drug, bacopa reversed the cognitive-dulling properties of the drug. Similarly, when bacopa was taken with the mood-regulator chlorpromazine, a drug similar to compazine, its effects were enhanced without any negative effects. Perhaps one of the most significant effect of bacopa is its ability to act as an adaptogen. Adaptogenic herbs are often rich in antioxidants and specifically aid in the ability of the person to handle and avoid damage from environmental stress. For these reasons, bacopa is an effective herb to treat people with AS that have extra difficulty with the ability to focus and retain a regular influx of information because of anxiety in the workplace or school.

Secondarily, it is helpful to treat or prevent ulcers, asthma, and prescription or illegal drug toxicity. Often standardized to 25 percent bacoside A, bacopa is given in amounts of 200–400 mg for the average person weighing approximately 150 pounds. In extract form, a common dose is 4–11 mL/day. In pill form, bacopa is more commonly found in combination with other herbs rather than as an isolated herb. Based on clinical experience, it works well in children as young as eight years old up to the elderly.

Chamomile (*Matricaria recutita*)

An old-fashioned herb used safely for hundreds of years, chamomile tea is best known to ease digestive discomfort of babies, children, and adults. Pharmalogical studies reveal the stalks, leaves, and flowers have both antispasmodic and sedative effects. Chamomile isn't as much for anxiety but irritability and insomnia. Typical doses for a 150 lb person are two teaspoons of dried herb for tea or two to three grams of capsules or tablets or 2–6 mL of tincture daily. Two common scenarios in which chamomile would really help is with a child or adult who gets stomachaches or is just plain irritable before school or work. For insomnia, it also works well with the person when having difficulty falling asleep, pounds the pillow and gets up muttering.

St. John's Wort (*Hypericum*)

I rarely use St. John's Wort or *Hypericum* to treat AS, and I find the people who have taken it before coming to my office have very mixed results. Despite its reputation as an antidepressant, St. John's Wort or *Hypericum* is better indicated for neuralgic pain like sciatica and stubbed toes. It seems to give inconsistent results and there are other herbs and amino acids that do a better job in reducing both anxiety and depression. Scientific research supports this, as the clinical trials are conflicting in their results. Even though St. John's Wort definitely shows anxiety-reducing effects, it tested considerably less effective than its conventional drug counterpart, benzodiazepines. Also, St. John's Wort interferes with the conventional medications such as citalopram (Celexa), nefazodone (Serzone), and, fluoxetine (Prozac).

ESSENTIAL FATTY ACIDS

About two-thirds of your brain consists of fatty acids. They are needed to build brain cells and to help brain cells allow nutrients in and out of the cells. Because the body can't manufacture two types, linoleic (LA) or omega-6 and alpha-linolenic acid (ALA) or omega-3, those two are called essential fatty acids. They must be obtained in the diet. Sources of ALA are flax seeds, chia seeds, walnuts, sea vegetables, green leafy vegetables, and coldwater fish such as salmon and tuna; while cold-pressed sunflower, safflower, corn, and sesame oils supply LA. Most people get adequate amounts of the LA essential fatty acid, but not the ALA.

ALA is further broken down into eicosapentaenoic acid (EPA), docosapentaenoic acid (DPA), and docosahexaenoic acid (DHA). DHA is the essential fatty acid most needed for brain function and intelligence. It raises dopamine, the neurotransmitter most involved with focus and motivation by 40% and has an antidepressant effect. In AS, when there is a deficiency of DHA we see an increase in the AD(H)D component of the condition. You can find DHA in small amounts in eggs and organ meats, but the most important sources are cold water seafood and algae. In fact, algae is where the fish get their source of DHA. In people with very healthy digestive systems, a certain amount of flax seed oil will convert to DHA. Therefore, supplementing with fish oils or with good quality algae if you are a vegetarian, would help with focus and AD(H)D.

While DHA will improve focus, EPA may help with depression. Many depressed patients have decreased EPA levels. In several British studies, researchers demonstrated that increasing EPA levels resulted in an antidepressant effect even in patients who had not responded well to conventional antidepressants.

Quality is very important because the fish oil companies vary in amounts of contaminants such as mercury or other toxic metals. Fish oils are concentrated foods. If the fish contains a certain percentage of mercury, its oil will contain even more. These toxic metals can cause a whole new set of problems for people with AS, which were discussed in Chapter 8. When purchasing fish oils, look for some assurance on the packaging that the product hãs been screened for mercury levels. While essential fatty acids are beneficial for many things, in the AS patient, I find them especially effective for all attention problems and for depression that doesn't respond to other treatment.

Even though amino acids, herbs, and essential fatty acids are potent medicines for anxiety and depression, I get faster results by also including constitutional homeopathy in my treatment plan.

CHAPTER 10

Homeopathy: A Giant Leap Forward

Another invaluable tool in treating Asperger Syndrome (AS) is the 200-year-old natural medical system called homeopathy. It originated in the late 1700s in Germany when a medical doctor named Samuel Hahnemann became concerned by the frequent occurrence of serious side effects from conventional drugs. Hahnemann researched and experimented with the use of dilute amounts of the drugs to minimize these effects. To his surprise, he found that the potency of the medicine was increased, while the side effects diminished. He then started studying both the conventional medical substances as well as dilute amounts of plants, minerals, and animals by testing them on healthy people. He discovered that each substance produced fairly consistent changes in the mental, emotional, and physical state of the test subjects. For example, *Mercurius* or mercury, a popular medicine in the 1850s, was used as a salve for syphilis. When Hahnemann tested dilute amounts on healthy volunteers, he discovered that fairly consistently, many would develop tremors, swollen lymph glands, sore throats with thick yellow-greenish discharge, a metallic taste in their mouths, would drool at night and become suspicious, anxious, socially withdrawn, mentally confused, and have morbid impulses that sometimes included harm to themselves or others. To explain this phenomenon, Hahnemann advanced the Law of Similars or, "Like Heals Like." According to Hahnemann, The Law of Similars states that, "a substance that produces a certain set of symptoms in a healthy person has the power to cure a sick person manifesting those same symptoms." After testing this theory and these medicines on hundreds of patients, he established a new form of medicine—constitutional homeopathy. Constitutional homeopathy is a dynamic medicine, which has continued to grow and become increasingly specific over the last 200 years. Currently, it is widely practiced in over eighty countries including all of Western and most of Eastern Europe, Russia, Mexico, the United States, and Canada. In Europe it is commonly prescribed by medical physicians either by itself or as an adjunct to conventional medicine.

In the United States, homeopathic medicine was taught in some conventional medical schools. Because of its success in the treatment of mental health conditions, several hospitals in the United States employing homeopathy were established including Hahnemann Hospital, now a conventional hospital in Philadelphia, Middletown (New York) State Homoeopathic Hospital, Menninger Clinic outside Topeka Kansas, and Homeopathic Hospital in New York City. As conventional medicines for mental health evolved, the time-consuming and very individualized homeopathy began playing a less significant role in this field. It takes fifteen to twenty minutes for a general practitioner to evaluate an anxious patient and prescribe a drug versus the often ninety minutes to find the correct remedy for the same person. In most cases the drug will effectively decrease the anxiety for as long as it is taken. The homeopathic remedy is nontoxic and works not only to treat the anxiety but also to rebalance the person. Most people report a "sense-of-well-being" after getting the correct homeopathic remedy and there is never that "drugged" feeling that can accompany conventional medications.

As with any form of medicine, the scientific community has studied homeopathy for decades. And while the debate marches on, scientific support has steadily gained momentum. A 1998 article in the prestigious medical journal, the *Lancet*, analyzed eighty-nine studies on homeopathy and concluded that it had a scientific effect beyond that of a placebo.[1] This reinforced the opinion of the 1991 article in the *British Medical Journal*. It stated that there was sufficient evidence to show that the results of homeopathy were positive.[2] More recently, the 2003 article in the *Pediatric Infectious Disease Journal* reviewed two randomized, controlled clinical trials of homeopathy in the treatment of childhood diarrhea, a significant source of childhood mortality in less developed countries.[3] The main author, Dr. Jacobs, confirmed that those children receiving homeopathic medicine recovered faster.

There is a recent resurgence in the United States due to increased awareness of the serious side effects, the cost of long-term treatment and the palliative rather than curative effect of many of these conventional medications. With this resurgence of homeopathy, there has been a flood of homeopathic products available to the consumer. Due to FDA (Federal Drug Administration) regulations, the labeling can be misleading. Often a vial of homeopathic medicine may say that it is appropriate for anxiety. And it is. But because there are many different types of anxiety and it can appear different from one person to the next, it's best to get advice on what to take from a provider who has studied homeopathy for many years. Additionally, there are many styles of homeopathy. The style that Hahnemann and ten generations of homeopathic physicians developed over 200 years is called constitutional or classical homeopathy. It brings the most long-term improvement to patients. Constitutional homeopathy is very individualized. The homeopathic doctor interviews each patient for one to two hours and develops a mental, emotional, and physical profile of that person. The doctor then matches that profile to one of over 1,000 well-studied homeopathic remedies. If chosen well, the remedy will rebalance the person mentally, emotionally, and physically.

Many physicians, like myself, joined the ranks of homeopathic doctors after challenging its validity. I started studying homeopathy when my mother-in-law became very ill. She has spent almost a year going from doctor to doctor with multiple diagnoses and trying various medicines. However, she grew weaker and weaker and eventually moved her bed down from her second-floor bedroom to the living room. This formerly very active woman was no longer able to even carry her laundry fifteen feet without having to stop and rest. She called me one day to tell me how, within a few months of trying homeopathic medicine, she was back on her feet and was out mowing her yard again. Certain that this was impossible, I starting studying homeopathy to explain to my mother-in-law how she was wasting her money on the ludicrous theory that by diluting a substance, it could increase its strength. After reading several books by leading constitutional homeopaths, I was intellectually intrigued but far from convinced. Unwilling to risk harming others, I tested it on myself, completely expecting it to make no change. Instead, it resolved the medical issue completely.

Since then, I have used homeopathy along with other natural medicines to treat conditions ranging from colds, to arthritis, to depression, to AS. I have found it to be gentle and effective. After diet, I consider it the most effective tool I have in treating AS. The following are four examples of the effectiveness of homeopathy in treating AS in both children and adults.

NELLIE, A 45-YEAR-OLD STAY-AT-HOME MOM

On the surface, Nellie seemed fine, a bit high-strung, but happy and functioning well. She had a twenty-year-marriage and was raising and home-schooling their four children. To the other home-schooling moms, Nellie was remarkably efficient, but a little distant. She really only made close friends with Mary, who also seemed a bit strange. The two of them rarely discussed anything that wasn't related to home-schooling. Nellie came to my office to treat her arthritis and sinus headaches that seem to be triggered by changes in the weather. Her knees felt stiff and cracked when descending stairs, and her left arm from shoulder to fingers had a tearing pain that was worse at night. She was forty-five and wanted an alternative to the conventional treatment of NSAIDs and more serious drugs. During the homeopathic intake, we discussed her family situation and her own mental and emotional state. She mentioned that her daughter had just been diagnosed with AS and that she herself must have something like ADHD as she could never remember a time when she just sat and did nothing. When Nellie discussed her anxiety, it was clear she had no idea how severe it was. Though she had a little trouble falling asleep because of her left arm pain, she woke every morning between four and six a.m. with anxious thoughts and heart palpitations. She could calm herself by praying and get back to sleep. She startled easily and became increasingly anxious when she had to leave the house and interact socially with others. It wasn't that she didn't feel capable; it was that she wasn't sure what she would say; or even worse, if she would either misinterpret what someone else said or say something herself that would unintentionally hurt another person's feelings. She tended to be extremely literal and seemed out-of-sync when communicating with others. In fact, communicating with others socially had never been easy for her. For example, she still flushed remembering the reaction of another mother when Nellie didn't agree that her child was an excellent swimmer. Nellie had competed in swimming as a child and teenager and knew the child had average ability at best. She didn't understand that the mother was really inviting a compliment, not a true assessment of the child's swimming proficiency.

In addition, I learned that Nellie loved cold milk, was allergic to cats, and had a lot of bloating after eating. Her arthritic pains and stiffness were always worse in the morning, and with the rain, and better after moving around a bit. She could temporarily relieve her arthritic pain and sinus headaches by extremely hot, almost scalding showers. Her dreams were action-packed as if she were watching a movie. And she frequently had swollen cervical glands.

It seemed apparent that Nellie has AS as well. Without telling her my suspicions, I suggested that she read a few books on the subject. She e-mailed me a few days later, surprised but relieved to finally understand the cause of her social deficiencies and anxiety.

The remedy that helped Nellie is called *Rhus toxicodendron* or the homeopathic version of poison ivy. It is a remedy that can benefit an anxious and restless person with arthritis that is worse in the morning and better with motion. It is also helpful with sinus conditions, and sleeplessness from anxiety. Nellie became nervous when she heard the plant basis of the remedy. When she was a child she had poison ivy so severely that her eyelids were swollen shut for three days and she was in bed for a week. Once assured she would not develop poison ivy from the medicine, she took the remedy and reported back three weeks later.

Her arthritic pain was about 80 percent better, but the real improvement for her was the decrease in anxiety. She no longer woke from anxiety and found herself less anxious in social settings. She still preferred the company of a single person or her own family, but the waves of anxiety were greatly diminished. In fact, she attended a home-school convention and felt significantly less anxious. She even turned and talked with the women on either side of her. Her sinus headaches were dramatically better and she was no longer painfully aware when the weather turned rainy. But the most telling change to me was her openness. She smiled more and was more relaxed.

Over the next two years, Nellie returned to my office every six to eight months to monitor her progress. She continued to improve over this period. It has been about three years since she last needed a dose of the remedy. Her anxiety is dramatically lessened and she wakes with anxiety only prior to extreme sources of uneasiness such as airline flights with four children, or cooking for the extended family during the holidays.

BRIAN, A THREE-YEAR-OLD GUY ON THE MOVE

At three-years-old, Brian was a handful. He had already been asked to leave three day cares for hitting the other children and having trouble settling down. His single mom, Sylvia, elected to quit her executive position, start a day care to help pay the bills, and look for solutions. The first thing she did was to get a diagnosis; Brian had AS. The therapist who made the diagnosis recommended conventional medications. The second thing Sylvia did was to bring Brian to my office.

Handing me the stack of psychological evaluations, Sylvia sat down and began to relate her son's medical history. He had trouble breast-feeding, then trouble with formula, followed by multiple ear infections and rounds of antibiotics leading to tubes in both ears. He alternated between diarrhea and constipation. Emotionally, Brian could be very aggressive. Sylvia noted that certain foods such as goldfish crackers would make him "go bonkers, run around completely hyper for an hour." He loved Chinese food but his behavior was worse after he ate it. In fact, his behavior was better when he didn't eat. Most of the time, his mom could calm him down by holding him very tightly and rocking him firmly. While he was in my office, he asked his mom to do this. But this was not always possible in public. Brian loved motion and was always on the go. He moved and talked a lot. He seemed extremely sensitive to the color "red." If he went to a store or home with a lot of red accents or if someone wore a bright red top or dress, he would become unhinged and be unable to calm down. Additionally, he was oversensitive in grocery stores and would run up and down the aisles. He had nightmares, swore a lot, and was overly fascinated with his genitals. He alternated between silliness and harming himself. He would ram his head into people and would deliberately burn himself with an iron and say, "it tickles." Finally, Brian liked to lick his mom, himself, and various objects. He seemed almost deliberate in his intent to behave inappropriately in public. Conversely, Brian could be incredibly sweet and affectionate with his mom and was quite bright.

Even though many AS children will share some of Brian's behaviors, they won't have them all. And that's where homeopathy can be so effective. By matching some of Brian's behaviors *that are not related to* AS with a remedy, both those and his AS behaviors can be reduced. In Brian's case, the correct remedy was *Hyoscyamus*. *Hyoscyamus* addresses the nervous system and is most appropriate for a person of any age who tends to swear, deliberately behaves inappropriately in public almost to shock others, talks a lot, is constantly moving and who has nightmares. It also contains typical AS behaviors such as oversensitivity to sound and color and decreased sensitivity to pain.

In addition to the remedy, I asked her to take sugar out of the house for a month, to eat organically, and avoid all food coloring, additives, and preservatives and to take a few other supplements. Despite Sylvia's eagerness to strictly comply with the program, we had a major stumbling block, Brian's dad. It had been a bitter divorce and custody battle. Brian lived with his mom for five days a week and with his dad on the weekends. His dad disputed the diagnosis, saying that there was nothing the matter with his son, and pretty much had no intention of adhering to a healthier diet.

Five weeks later, a smiling Brian and Sylvia entered the office to report back in. It was an amazing difference in behavior. He had decreased hitting others or himself and was less aggressive overall. His sensory issues were diminished. He could see the color "red" without becoming hyper. He stopped burning himself on the iron or ramming his head into people. Sylvia no longer saw the excessive silliness. Much calmer overall, Brian was now able to go food shopping and even Christmas shopping for several hours without any emotional meltdowns. Even biting others, a symptom not mentioned at the first visit had decreased. Physically, he no longer vacillated between constipation and diarrhea and hadn't had any nightmares since the remedy. The only time that Brian wasn't stable was Sunday evening and Monday morning after he visited his father where he received sugar and food additives. In addition, Sylvia realized that Brian also was sensitive to certain fragrances in hand creams and soaps as well as air fresheners and now kept them out of the house. One year later, Brian is still doing well and is now happily attending a regular preschool.

TOM, A THIRTY-FIVE-YEAR-OLD COMPUTER ENGINEER

At first glance, it was hard to see that Tom had AS. Though soft-spoken, he was cordial and started out with a little small talk. He had a good job in a medium-sized company with a lot of responsibility. As long as he could remember, he had anxiety issues. Anxiety seemed to run in his family, so it was something he considered natural. It wasn't until after he married eight years ago that he realized his thought pattern and nervous system were dramatically different from most people. When he was anxious, he would hold his body very tightly, which was a peculiar stance to others. He was oversensitive to sounds, like air conditioning or paddle fans, or the sound of fluorescent lights and smells. He overreacted with anger to minor things like having to replace a busted light bulb and didn't react to other things like falling, getting a cut, and bleeding profusely while hiking. Tom also had some obsessive-compulsive tendencies. A good cook, he liked the kitchen utensils in a particular order and couldn't start to cook unless things were just right. He would also write out lists for everything. For example, when they went on a trip to the coast, he wrote down all the items he needed to pack or bring—despite the fact it was just a weekend trip two hours from home. However, the real reason he came into my office was his marriage. Initially, his wife joked about his extreme need for routine, solitude, obsessive-compulsive tendencies, and overreactivity. But over the years, he realized it was wearing on her. They were less physically intimate. She would ask if there was a problem and he would just say no. How could he tell her that no matter how much he loved her, he didn't have the same level libido that she did and sometimes it really bugged him to be touched by anyone—especially someone who was hot and smelling of sweat. But that was only part of the problem. Never a particularly social person, even less so with the stress of his job, he found himself more and more reluctant to do things on the weekend that involved other people. His wife was starting to do things with others on her own. He began to worry that she was planning to divorce him and he didn't want to be alone.

Physically, Tom slept poorly and would often have night sweats, despite being a bit on the chilly side. He would get discomfort from gas and was frequently constipated. He tended to have repeated bouts of jock itch under his arms and in his groin, as well as athlete's foot. As a child he had ear infections accompanied by multiple rounds of antibiotics. In addition, he had mild scoliosis and occasionally suffered from abscesses. He had a bad reaction to a recent tetanus vaccination. Tom was most concerned that I help him "be normal" so his wife wouldn't leave him.

The homeopathic remedy that helped Tom is called *Silica*. *Silica* works well in anxious, sensitive, chilly people who have a tendency toward fungal infections and night sweats. They have many insecurities and need to write lists as a form of control over their own chaos. They also tend to have some artistic component in their lives. In Tom's case, it was ethnic cooking.

One month later, Tom returned to my office, this time with his wife, Sherry. Since the remedy and the marriage counseling that I also recommended, they were doing better. She read a book on AS and stopped taking Tom's behavior personally. Instead, she suggested Saturdays be Tom's day and Sunday be a day they would do things together. They were still working out the sexual intimacy concerns. But as Sherry commented, "We need to work on this just like other marriages need to work on one spouse having a condition like diabetes. Tom is still hardworking, honest, and a good provider." Besides, as Sherry was candid enough to point out, she had trouble her whole life with compulsive eating and Tom had never said a negative word.

ELLEN, ON THE BRINK OF ADULTHOOD, BUT NOT MOVING FORWARD

Ellen blinked nervously at me, as she walked into my office, ushered by her mom. She was a twenty-year-old young woman who seemed incredibly healthy and full of energy.

Ellen had been really looking forward to college. Her supportive parents enrolled her in a small college about thirty miles from home. She was excited about moving into a dorm and hoped to move past the unpleasant memories of high school. This was her big chance to prove she was just like everyone else. Two months later, she returned home, defeated. There wasn't enough structure at the college to keep her focused and the social aspects were overwhelming. Just living with someone who liked scented candles and hated the quiet had been difficult. But trying to study in a library instead of her comfortable bedroom had led to several outbursts that frightened both her roommate and the other people in her dorm. In one outburst, she started to growl, while in another, she hid under her desk, rocking. Finally, the college suggested that Ellen might not be ready either emotionally or academically.

As a young child, Ellen had multiple ear infections and the corresponding antibiotics. She preferred to sit and watch the school and day care personnel during naptime and rarely joined in play with the other children. Over the years, she had tried many conventional drugs. Some she reacted to right away; others worked well for a while and then stopped. Currently, she was taking Risperidone for her blinking tic, citalopram for the depression, and time-released methylphenidate for her hyperactivity.

Ellen had a fairly good diet with fruits, vegetables, whole grains, and meat. She especially loved cottage cheese and lemons. She would eat lemons the way others eat oranges. Ellen also had a sweet tooth and was extremely thirsty, especially for cold water.

In addition to her AS symptoms, Ellen also suffered from pounding headaches. These pounding headaches came on suddenly and were so intense that she needed to retreat into a quiet room away from others where she would moan and punch her pillow.

Ellen came to my office to find a means to reduce her medications and to return to college. Her mom was there to support Ellen in this process. At any age, family support is helpful, but in children and young adults, it is the key to the success of the treatment. They help the person maintain the program on a daily basis.

The remedy I chose for Ellen was *Belladonna*. *Belladonna* works well in patients who look extremely healthy, have pounding headaches that come on quickly, are sensitive to noise and light, like lemons and who may make animal noises when angry. I also recommended that she withdraw sugar from the diet for thirty days.

One month later, Ellen returned to my office with a big smile. Her blinking was gone! She was also more able to talk about her anger and had fewer outbursts. As often happens during the second visit, the patient gives me a clearer idea of the intensity of the condition. In this case, Ellen admitted that she used to scratch other people when she got angry. That had also stopped during this month. The debilitating headaches had gone away. Interestingly, she now seemed to have more obsessive-compulsive behaviors. I find that when one major behavior pattern subsides, an underlying one surfaces. I told her to be patient with this change, as it would gradually decrease as well.

Now, under the direction of her prescribing physician, Ellen was ready to start decreasing her conventional medications. Over the next three months, the medications were slowly but steadily decreased. After the third month, Ellen was off the citalopram and had cut the Risperidone and methylphenidate in half.

All was going wonderfully for about five months. Then Ellen's mom sent an urgent e-mail—Ellen was reverting back to the outbursts and growling. A few days later in my office, the whole story came out. Ellen had been ill with chest congestion and had used a strong-smelling menthol rub for a few days. Within a few days, her behavior deteriorated and her sugar cravings took over. I gave her another dose of the remedy and she promised to avoid sugar and to come back and see me in a month.

Ellen looked radiant as she entered the office. She had been doing extremely well and had just returned from a visit to the college. She was returning to school in the summer, as a trial, and would be getting her own room in the dorm. The last I heard from her mom, Ellen was doing wonderfully, still needed 0.25 mg of Risperidone daily and had discovered that daily exercise and avoiding sugar allowed her to go off the methylphenidate completely.

What we have described are four very different cases. Each person has AS, but with unique presentations. Each person's physical symptoms varied as well and therefore, each person required a different homeopathic remedy. Homeopathy is so effective because of its specificity. There is a single remedy that will be appropriate for most situations.

Despite its effectiveness, homeopathy is not a panacea. The homeopathic practitioner must study intensively for many years and be extremely observant and ask the right questions. In addition, the practitioner must have a working knowledge of at least 400 out of the 1000+ different homeopathic remedies and be able to recognize each remedy in both male and female, and in youth, middle age, and old age. For his part, the patient must avoid some commonplace substances in order to avoid antidoting or stopping the action of the homeopathic remedy: some of these substances are coffee, menthol, and birth control pills. It can be difficult to avoid these substances. For example, prior to homeopathy, Nellie enjoyed a daily cup of coffee. She antidoted her remedy three times the first year in her effort to see if the coffee exclusion didn't apply to her. Each time she antidoted the remedy, her anxiety and arthritic pain returned. Finally, she decided that it was worth giving up coffee for decreased anxiety and pain-free joints. In children, it's often antibiotics that undermine the homeopathic remedy. Many parents are often not even aware that there are many natural, effective, and safe alternatives to antibiotics to treat all sorts of infections including ear and sinuses. These natural medicines work best when taken at the first sign of illness.

Each remedy can be sensitive to different things. For some, coffee isn't a problem, but mint is. It can take six months to a couple of years for a remedy to hold without further doses. Despite these limitations, most people think that it is well worth the avoidance of these substances to be effectively treated with a medicine that has no long-term adverse effect and doesn't require daily requirement of pills. A complete list of antidoting factors is in the Appendix.

The typical first visit takes between one and a half and two hours. It can take between one and three times to get the correct remedy. Each person on a remedy must learn to recognize what it's doing and when it stops. If the remedy stops working or the person changes to a different remedy, a return visit is needed. The patient may need three to four visits that first year to get the desired results. Homeopathy is economical, but necessitates the active cooperation of the patient. The better the patient understands himself or his child, the more favorable the outcome.

When looking for a homeopathic physician, ask what kind of homeopathy they practice. If they don't say either constitutional or classical homeopathy, then the medicine isn't addressing the entire person and is generally less effective and must be repeated more often.

To get a better idea of how classical homeopathy works in treating Asperger Syndrome, these two books are especially helpful: A *Drug-Free Approach to Asperger Syndrome and Autism* by Judyth Reichenberg-Ullman, Robert Ullman, and Ian Luepker and the *Impossible Cure* by Amy Lansky.

While using homeopathy for treating minor illnesses is very safe, please be extremely cautious about treating Asperger Syndrome in yourself or your child with homeopathy. The incorrect remedy can make behavior, anxiety, and mood worse in some people. If done once or twice, the effect passes within a few days. If multiple homeopathic remedies are used incorrectly, the person can become worse. It takes many years of study and clinical practice to correctly prescribe most effect remedy out of hundreds of common remedies.

WHAT TO EXPECT

When a correct homeopathic remedy is given, the person feels more balanced. Sometimes that concerns those around the person. For example, a young man who tended to keep his feelings to himself and be fairly complacent with his parents and at school received a remedy. He started expressing his own opinions to his parents. In fact, he refused to go out birdwatching with his parents as he never enjoyed it. His parents initially interpreted this as misbehavior. However, when he was able to articulate his feelings and needs at school, they quickly saw that while a complacent child is easier to raise, it's also helpful to know how to assert yourself.

Homeopathy can't make a person change their basic nature, but it can soften it. For example, an affectionate but impulsive child will still keep their happy nature but decrease their impulsivity. Similarly, a quiet person fixated on his job will still be quiet, but may now be able to better participate in a conversation about other topics. Most people tell me that they feel like they can handle stress better and have dramatically less anxiety.

While everything in this book will help, I find that diet and homeopathy cause the greatest and quickest gains.

CHAPTER 11

What You Can Do Right Now

There are no two identical cases of Asperger Syndrome (AS). Even though each case will have social awkwardness, anxiety, overreactivity, arriving at incorrect conclusions, sensory issues and literalness, each person has different ways of showing these same characteristics. Some will also have prosopagnosia (face blindness), or topographic agnosia (place blindness). Some will have auditory processing dysfunction. Others will have sound sensitivity, but not be noise or taste sensitive. Because of this, each case is most successfully treated separately as what works for one may not work for another. There is no magic bullet in the treatment of AS in either conventional or natural medicine. Instead, it's an individualized combination of treatments that seems to really help. On the top of that list is diet and everything that was discussed in Chapter 7. This is something you can do at home at very little cost. Make the dietary changes for at least one month. However, there are many other beneficial things you can consider as adjuncts to a medical treatment plan. Not everyone will benefit from each of these recommendations, but everyone will benefit from a few. If something works, incorporate it into your or your child's lifestyle.

1. Yoga—Yoga is a repetitive form of exercise that, with its simple breathing techniques, calms the nervous system and may decrease the anxiety and improve overall mood. It also gives the frequently awkward AS persons a better awareness of their body and may increase coordination. The 2006 article entitled, "Effect of Yoga Based Lifestyle Intervention on State and Trait Anxiety," by Gupta describes the anxiety-reducing effects of a ten-day yoga immersion in test subjects both with anxiety disorders and without.[1] Another study by researchers Michalsen et al. in the *Medical Science Monitor*, demonstrated that a three-month program

for a group of twenty-four women who perceived themselves as "mentally distressed" resulted in not only a decrease in the anxiety but also in physical complaints.[2] The *British Journal of Sports Medicine* reviewed the research on yoga and anxiety and concluded, "owing to the diversity of conditions treated and poor quality of most of the studies, it is not possible to say that yoga is effective in treating anxiety or anxiety disorders in general. However, there are encouraging results, particularly with obsessive compulsive disorder."[3] University of California researchers Woolery et al. studied the effects of yoga on twenty-eight young participants with self-diagnosed mild depression. "Subjects who participated in the yoga course demonstrated significant decreases in self-reported symptoms of depression and trait anxiety. ... Changes also were observed in acute mood, with subjects reporting decreased levels of negative mood and fatigue following yoga classes."[4] These and many more studies support the use of yoga in the treatment of anxiety. Yoga programs are readily available including some specific for children with AS.

2. Brain Gym—Brain Gym is a specific technique that physical and occupational therapists use. Using physical movement to enhance mental ability, it facilitates better communication between the two sides of the brain in relationship to the body. Developed in the late 1970s by educators Drs. Paul Dennison and Gail Dennison, it is gaining recognition in thousands of schools, corporations, and athletic programs throughout eighty countries and may be a helpful tool with some people, especially those more physically challenged with AS.

3. Color Therapy—While the use of color isn't usually considered a medical treatment, hospitals routinely use blue fluorescent lights for jaundiced newborns, and colored fluorescent lights are also used as an adjunct in conditions such as chronic myeloid leukemia. Whole industries use color as a tool to influence people. The use of color in advertisements, or in new pharmaceutical medication, clothing, and interior design is commonplace. And while the scientific basis of the effects of color on people hasn't been clearly determined, what is clear is that it can have a definitive effect. Similarly, it can be a helpful adjunct in AS. Colors can be stimulating, calming, or neutral. For example, some of my AS patients have mentioned how they avoid a large box store that features the color bright red. They become agitated within a few minutes of entering the store. Others mentioned that they have trouble with certain computer background colors. They feel unsettled or agitated with some colors, but not with others. Often there is a sensory overload. And while many aren't consciously even aware of these nuances, they will commonly wear very bland colors for clothing.

The use of calming colors can be extended to the home. Often cooler colors like the blues and greens or soft cheerful colors are best. Skeptical, one of my patients repainted her living room to a soft but sunny yellow. She found that she began spending more and more time in that room.

So, if you have a child with AS, please choose a calming color for their bedroom. If you are an adult with AS, look at your home. Which rooms are you most comfortable in and which are more unsettling? If your bedspread is a harsh color, consider a softer or cooler color.

4. Create a sanctuary, not a hermitage—both the adult and the child having AS need a place to decompress from the overreactivity and anxiety. While a room would be ideal, this place should be small, with little to no sensory stimulating colors or objects, and should be private. One AS teen would lie down behind the sofa after school. He wanted quiet time to destress away from his non-AS brothers. Another, when weather permitted, would seek out a very large weeping willow tree and hide in the little room its dangling branches created. A third teen had a window box complete with curtains to retreat to. Being able to center oneself in a safe place is crucial for maintaining a calm home. But a sanctuary is different from a hermitage. It's not healthy to allow an AS child to close out others for long periods of time.

5. Music Therapy—The medical field has studied the effects of music on everything from treating multiple sclerosis, to surgical recuperation, to treating anxiety and depression. The majority of the studies suggest that music is consistently beneficial. Anecdotally, some AS symptoms such as anxiety and depression respond well to music. Interestingly, no one type of music seems to help. Some seem to gravitate toward hard rock, while others lean toward classical music. In one patient, classical music made her angry and irritated. Consider the desired psychological effect. If it's to calm, then find music that has a tempo similar to a restful heart rate of between sixty-five and seventy-five beats per minute.

6. Meditation—Meditation is a restful state in which the person is fully alert mentally and physically. According to a 2005 article in the *International Journal of Psychophysiology*, researchers Takahashi et al. studied the effects of meditation on EEG readings.[5] Their results show that meditation increases the parasympathetic (calming restorative state) and decreases the sympathetic (fight or flight) portions of the autonomic nervous system.

   Meditation is a somewhat controversial subject among people with AS. Some say that it increases their anxiety rather than diminish it. A 2003 article in *Depression and Anxiety* by NIMH researchers Tsao and Craske gives one explanation. Those with anxiety worse at night demonstrated increased panic and anxiety during a meditation exercise compared to those with daytime anxiety. Tsao and Craske suggest that, "nocturnal panic individuals fear situations that involve a loss of vigilance (e.g., relaxation, fatigue, and altered states of consciousness)."[6]

7. Biofeedback—A method that is very helpful for treating many anxiety-related aspects of AS, biofeedback uses electronic monitoring of hand temperature or muscle tension to train people how to relax. The person

learns to voluntarily monitor and control body functions such as heart rate, blood pressure, muscle contractions, and brain waves. During a biofeedback session, the person will have electrodes attached to various parts of the body to monitor neural and muscular changes. A series of lights or beeps relay these changes to the person. For example, as the hands become colder or the muscles tense, the beeps would accelerate, signaling to the person to adapt a more relaxed posture. It's a process of trial-and-error until the person learns with the help of the biofeedback administrator, how to control the anxiety. This process requires several sessions of training, but then once the training has been incorporated by the person, he recognizes the physical symptoms related to anxiety and can relax on his own.

8. Support Groups—Another resource that works well for some people are support groups. Both AS adult and children groups are divided into two main types: professionally or peer-led. Professionally led support groups are facilitated by a mental health specialist, often a social worker or psychologist, and tend to work on social and communication skills. Peer-led are less formal and focus on providing a supportive environment for like-minded people to feel completely at ease. There is often a sense of self-validation to look around at AS peers and see many successful professionals in the group. Peer-led groups tend to be more social in nature and are available in all major cities and in many colleges. AS children's support groups are especially helpful during the various childhood transitions. The groups tend to cover a limited age span such as preteens, teenagers, or post-high school young adults. The groups help the child see that there are others with similar thought and behavioral patterns and give a safe environment to practice skills that would help them at a particular age adapt to the non-AS world.

9. Special Interest Groups, both online and local unrelated to AS—A more recent phenomenon are local online meet groups. For example, many AS people take advantage of small, six to eight-person group, hikes for which they sign up online, show up at the meet point, hike to a destination, and then return. There is a certain instant camaraderie, which spontaneously happens, and which allows the AS person to avoid awkward silences. Unusual behavior is better tolerated. A friend told me about an online hiking group that she had joined. As she was describing and naming the seven other people in the group, I realized one was an AS patient of mine. All she said was that he was a bit quiet, but nice, and wore a dress shirt and long pants on the first hike, but returned the following week with normal hiking clothes. Others do the same with book clubs, art clubs, etc. The functions are driven by a common interest and meetings have a purpose rather than being strictly social. Since there is no focus on AS, it's a great way to socialize in a safe environment. Make sure that the groups are part of a larger structure rather than a person posting for hiking buddies on some Internet list.

10. Camps, lessons, and clubs for children—There are some wonderful alternative camps that are cropping up all over the country including some geared for kids more affected by AS. They offer the usual fare of outdoor activities and arts and crafts, but with a staff sensitive to the needs of this community.

11. Occupational Therapists for adults—In Chapter 4 there was a description of what occupational therapists do. If you think of occupational therapists as trying to help you do your job at home or in the workplace better, you can see that there are many applications, such as sensory issues, in which an OT would help.

12. Anger Management Books or Courses—There are some good courses and books for those with anger management problems. Since having poor recognition of emotions can be part of the AS picture, sometimes the child and especially the adult isn't even aware that he is having angry outbursts. He will think that he is simply expressing his point-of-view. These books are a discrete way for a professional to learn to control a trait that works against healthy personal and professional relationships. I have included some titles in the Appendix.

13. Acting—One of the most effective means to learn speaking and social skills for both children and adults is through acting. If the AS child learns this from an early age, it will be extremely beneficial for his whole life. Many young adults have similar benefits from acting classes at community/college level. Inherent in the acting class setting is both a tolerance for mistakes and a focus on elocution and delivery. One successful middle-aged woman with AS recounted years of mini-plays performed in her family. Even though she was the "quiet" child, her mother gently insisted on her participation knowing that the enthusiastic audience feedback would positively reinforce the experience. When she reached high school and beyond, she had overcome the paralyzing fear of being in front of others. Another middle-aged man with AS, who seemed completely at ease in formal settings, shared that he spent years developing this social confidence in community theatre. In a condition that frequently includes low self-esteem, this can be an effective tool to counter that. This ability to temporarily sidestep the severe anxiety by maintaining an acting posture will help the individual both personally and professionally. An amusing example of this is a wonderful Christopher Walkens' movie entitled, *Who Am I This Time?* in which he plays a gifted actor who has many Asperger-like symptoms offstage.

14. Art Therapy—Just as it sounds, art therapy is using many artistic mediums such as paint, sand, crayons, and collage to help the child with expression, sensory issues, and communication. This can be done in the school setting or at the therapist's office.

15. Facilitated Social Skills and Organizational Training—Often offered by therapists or former special education teachers, these coaches emphasize

social and organizational skills for both children and adults through discussion, roleplaying and other activities. This happens in both one-on-one and group sessions. This is especially important when the adult or child's lack of social skills has become detrimental to the person. The value in these groups is that the participants see that there are others with the same condition and that they can make mistakes in a safe, nonthreatening environment.

Here is a small example of how a coach can help. An AS professor tended to stumble with holiday questions. When asked, "Are you doing anything special over the Christmas holiday?" he would answer literally and often inappropriately, "I have kids in college and can't afford to go do anything as all my disposable income goes toward their tuition. I also have a journal article that needs to be written. And, I'm not a Christian and don't celebrate Christmas." The person asking would hastily retreat. One even said as he backed away, "That was way more information than I needed." The coach helped the professor give friendly generic answers to his colleagues and just as importantly, to understand that the question is just a conversational tool.

There are multiple social nuances that many, though not all, people with AS tend to be oblivious to. It sometimes helps to have someone other than a family member to get some direction. Again, most children and adults thrive in these groups and others do not. When persons with AS have a supportive home environment and trust a parent or spouse to guide them in more challenging social arenas, then these groups may be unnecessary. There are dozens of unfacilitated social groups around the country of successful professional adults with AS that provide a similar function. The benefit to these groups is that they frequently reinforce the positive aspects of AS and nurture the less adept members of the Asperger community.

16. Speech and Language Therapy—Another therapy that is more directed at children, the Speech and Language Therapy, addresses both the characteristic monotone voice of AS and the difficulty with communication. This includes helping the child learn how to initiate and maintain a conversation as well as understand body language and facial expressions.

17. College Classes and Social Skills—Many community colleges offer non-credit courses in conversational skills. These classes are often targeted toward those in the computer or other more technical industries that have trouble with coworkers or even starting and maintaining a simple conversation

GENERAL ADVICE FOR RAISING YOUR AS CHILD

One of the most important things to understand is that AS doesn't just happen; it's a behavior and thought pattern that was passed on to your child—most likely genetically. I have yet to meet an AS child whose parents didn't have some aspect of AS behavior—whether AD(H)D-like behavior, OCD tendencies, or anxiety. Sadly, many of these parents completely deny these behaviors even when they are extremely obvious. Please don't think of your child as defective or as needing to be fixed or cured. Sure, the child needs to adapt to a non-AS world, but some Asperger symptoms such as attention to detail, loyalty, long-term fascination with a single topic, if channeled correctly, can be very productive in a successful career. Having a limited personal social life is not a handicap; but not being about to interact socially or to network when needed is.

Don't bully your AS child. It won't work. The person with AS often has rigid ideas and must be persuaded through patient logic rather than force. Some parents joke that their children redefine the word "stubborn." I've heard accounts of AS teens arguing for hours without conceding a point even while privileges were being taken away. Instead, the parents with successful well-adjusted AS children work on building the self-esteem. Persons who feel good about themselves put up fewer boundaries and have more confidence to venture into more challenging situations. The most successful parents start very early and find some area in which their child can be competent or excel, whether it is music, sports, writing, carpentry, or photography. Photography or writing skills can help the reserved AS high school student get on the school newspaper. Carpentry skills will be welcome in the theatre department. If someone is skilled, poor social skills are often tolerated. Start sports at a very young age. It will not only help with gross motor coordination but will also provide a means for the child to interact with other children. The reason to start it early is that many AS children have poor coordination and will have a tougher time becoming proficient if they learn casually in school or have their first exposure on a team setting.

Computer gaming typically doesn't count as a social interaction. Be careful to limit this unless there is some direct social involvement. During high school, because of his computer skills, one AS teen was frequently invited to LAN (local area network) parties, in which a group of kids bring their computers to one home and play gaming marathons. This is not the same as strangers talking with each other over the Internet without any face-to-face contact. It's never too early to teach AS children to successfully interact with others. The best types of interactions are those planned around a function such as Boy Scouts or 4-H. These are small groups of kids that are closely supervised by adults. There are AS teen camps in many states that offer a supportive environment. They are supervised by adults who understand the challenges of the AS population.

A pitfall that many well-meaning parents fall into is throwing everything at the child at once to "fix" the problem. Based on my experience with this population, often the most effective things cost little to no money. An affluent parent made this comment, "I could afford to try anything and everything for my child. So, I did. My friend couldn't. My child is not better off than hers despite all the programs."

A FEW WORDS IN CLOSING

Asperger Syndrome has probably always existed in a milder form. Food alterations and increase in airborne pollutants have contributed to its increased intensity. This book offers a gentler way to decrease that intensity. It also suggests a different way to look at this condition. It is our sincere hope that this will lead you or your child to a happier and more fulfilled life.

Resources Helpful in Addressing Asperger Syndrome

TO CONTACT DR. LAWTON'S OFFICE FOR MORE INFORMATION ON ASPERGER SYNDROME

The Lawton Clinic – 503-443-2332
www.aspergerbook.com

COMPANIES AND SERVICES USEFUL FOR TREATING ASPERGER SYNDROME

The following is a list of companies who provide products or services that may be helpful in the process of decreasing the intensity of AS. While your natural physician may suggest some excellent alternatives, you can find most of these products locally or on the Internet. In my experience, there are many large companies whose product quality is marginal and some small local companies, which have excellent quality products. As emphasized throughout the book, the better the quality of the product or services, the better and more consistent the results.

GOOD COMPANIES YOU CAN FIND AT YOUR LOCAL HEALTH FOOD STORE

Enzymedica (http://www.enzymedica.com)—Offers a wide range of enzymes including ones that break down the cell walls of candida albicans.
Gaia Herbs—Quality herbal company

Jarrow—sells Luo Han Sweet, a natural sweetener in powder form.

New Chapter—A full spectrum of products including enzymes and probiotics.

Newayceuticals—Sells the whole fruit sweetener, Luo Han Guo, as a syrup.
While this product may soon be available in stores, it is currently available
online at http://www.newayceutical.com/Merchant2/merchant.mvc?

Wise Woman Herbal Products—Quality herbal company

LABORATORIES

Most of these laboratories require a doctor's signature to run a test. However,
you may want to provide this contact information to your physician.

Analytical Research Labs, Inc.—Hair analyses screening for 20 minerals
and toxic chemicals.
2225 W. Alice Avenue
Phoenix, Arizona 85021 USA
1-602-995-1580
http://www.arltma.com

Bio-Center Lab—Tests for pyroluria
3100 N Hillside
Wichita, KS 67219
800-494-7785 or 316-684-7784
http://biocenterlab.org/

Direct Health Care Access II Lab, Inc.—Tests for pyroluria
350 W. Kensington Road Suite 107
Mount Prospect, IL 60056 847-222-9546
http://info@pyroluriatesting.com
http://www.pyroluriatesting.com/

Doctor's Data, Inc.—Digestion and heavy metal testing
3755 Illinois Avenue, St.
Charles, IL 60174
Phone (800) 323-2784 or (630) 377-8139, Fax (630) 587-7860
http://www.doctorsdata.com

Genova Diagnostics Laboratory—Digestion and heavy metal testing
PO Box 3220
Asheville, NC, 28802-3220
Toll free phone: 1-866-210-8039
Fax: 1-828-232-1364
http://www.gdx.net/home/

Great Plains Lab—Digestion and heavy metal testing
11813 West 77th
Lenexa, KS 66214
913-341-8949
913-341-6207 fax
http://gpl4u@aol.com
http://www.greatplainslaboratory.com/

Trace Elements, Incorporated—Hair analysis
4501 Sunbelt Drive
Addison, Texas 75001 USA
Toll Free 1 (800) 824-2314
Phone: (972) 250-6410 Fax: (972) 248-4896
http://www.traceelements.com/

U.S. Biotek—IgG and IgE screening for diet, environmental toxins and
    allergens
13500 Linden Ave
North Seattle, WA 98133 USA
Phone: 1.877.318.8728 Fax: 206.363.8790
http://www.usbiotek.com/

BOOKS ON HOMEOPATHY AS RELATED TO ASPERGER SYNDROME AND AUTISM SPECTRUM CONDITIONS

A Drug-Free Approach to Asperger Syndrome and Autism. Judyth
Reichenberg-Ullman, Robert Ullman, and Ian Luepker. Edmonds, WA:
Picnic Point Press, 2005.
An Impossible Cure. Amy L. Lansky. Portola Valley, CA: R. L. Ranch Press,
2003.

BOOKS ON ASPERGER SYNDROME AND BULLYING

Perfect Targets: Asperger Syndrome and Bullying. R. Heinrichs. Shawnee
Mission, KS: Autism Asperger Publishing Company, 2003.
Asperger Syndrome and Bullying. Nick Dubin. London: Jessica King Publish-
ing, 2007.

BOOKS ON AMINO ACID THERAPY

The Edge Effect. E. R. Braverman. New York: Sterling Publishing Co., 2004.
Depression-Free, Naturally. Joan Mathews Larson. New York: Ballantine
Publishing Group, 1999.
The Brain Chemistry Diet. Michael Lesser. New York: G. P. Putnam's Sons,
2002.

COOKBOOKS

Eating Well for Optimal Health. Andrew Weil. New York: Knoph, 2000.
The Healthy Kitchen: Recipes for a Better Life, Body and Spirit. Andrew Weil.
  New York: Knoph, 2002.
Stealth Health: How to Sneak Nutrition Painlessly into your Diet. Evelyn Tri-
  bole. New York: Penguin Group, 2000.

ENVIRONMENTALLY FRIENDLY PAINTS

EcoSpec®
Introduced in 1994 by Benjamin Moore Paints, and featuring very low
  volatile organic compounds (VOCs), EcoSpec® paint meets the most
  stringent environmental requirements. As an acrylic paint for interior
  use, it is virtually odorless and unusually quick drying, so rooms can be
  used immediately after being painted.

Safe Coat by AFM
http://www.afmsafecoat.com/. In business since the 1980s, AFM remains
  the only company to provide a complete range of chemically responsible
  building and maintenance products.

Dulux Lifemaster Paint—made with no added VOC and available at ICI
  paint stores http://www.icipaintstores.com/.

SITES ON FACE-BLINDNESS AND PLACE-BLINDNESS

http://www.prosopagnosia.com/main/likewhat/index.asp
  Cecilia Burman—A very informative site by a person with prosopagnosia.
http://www.choisser.com/faceblind/—This is an Internet book on Face
  Blindness written by a person with prosopagnosia. Many chapters of
  this book are excellent; however, the writer's personal angst pervades
  other sections.
http://www.faceblind.org/—Harvard and University College in London
  prosopagnosia researcher, Bradley Duchaine's authoritative site on face
  blindness.
http://www.newhorizons.org/spneeds/inclusion/teaching/stockdale.html
  topographic agnosia

APPENDIX B

Common Mercury Derivatives

SYNONYMS FOR THIMEROSOL

http://www.hgtech.com/Information/Thimerosal.htm. Though mercury toxic exposure is primarily airborne, look for these mercury derivatives in hair color, over-the-counter antiseptics, cosmetics, and other products around the house.

(1, 2)-(O-Carboxyphenyl)thio) ethyl mercury sodium salt; Elcide 75; Elicide; Ethyl (2-mercaptobenzoato-S) mercury sodium salt; O-(Ethylmercurithio) benzoic acid sodium salt; Ethylmercurithiosalicylic acid sodium salt; Ethylmerkurithiosalicilan Sodny (Czech); Ethyl (sodium O-ercaptobenzoato) mercury; Mercurothiolate; Mercury, Ethyl (2-Mercaptobenzoate-S)-, sodium salt; Merfamin; Merthiolate; Merthiolate salt; Merthiolate sodium; Mertorgan; Merzonin; Merzonin sodium; Merzonin, sodium salt; SET; Sodium Ethylmercuric Thiosalicylate; Sodium O-(ethylmercurithio) benzoate; Sodium Ethylmercurithiosalicylate; Sodium Merthiolate; Thimerosalate; Thimerosol; Thimersalate; Thiomerosal; Thiomersal; Thiomersalate

Tasty Pesto Recipes Which Will Also Help with Chemical Detoxification

PESTO

I'm always suggesting that people use food rather than pills to treat AS. Foods are absorbed better, are less expensive, and contain a wider range of beneficial nutrients than pills. One of my favorite discoveries is fresh organic pesto. Though I have always enjoyed fresh pesto over my pasta, Dr. Joyce Young first introduced me to pesto as an immune booster, digestive aid, and liver cleanser a few years ago. I'm including several different ways to prepare the fresh pesto. And no, packaged pesto in the stores is not the same; it must be fresh and organic. In fact, whenever any food in this Appendix is mentioned, just assume that it has the word organic in front of it, so I don't have to keep repeating it.

Also, I am much more concerned with you eating herbs than following recipes exactly. If you sample a herb and don't like the taste, then don't use it. Or if you don't like garlic or you want extra cheese, go ahead. Just don't forget to include the herbs.

Pesto can be any combination of the following herbs:

Arugala—goes well in small amounts directly in salads
Basil
Chives
Cilantro
Dill
Lemon grass
Marjoram (tastes similar to oregano)
Mint
Oregano

Parsley (Italian is somewhat higher in nutrition than the curly)
Rosemary—traditionally used for increased brain function, it's strong-tasting so use it in moderation.
Sage

Ways to Incorporate Fresh Organic Herbs into Your Diet

Pesto over Spaghetti

This same recipe can go over grilled chicken or fish after it has been cooked:

Ingredients:

1 Large bunch of ultra-fresh basil (1 cup after finely mincing)
¼ bunch parsley (optional)
1–2 large garlic cloves, very finely sliced, and then minced
½ cup organic walnuts or pine nuts
Half cup very finely diced organic sun-dried tomatoes, preferably oil packed (don't put in if making this for children as they tend not to like sun-dried tomatoes)
¼ cup grated organic Parmesan cheese
2 tbsp extra virgin olive oil (optional)

Directions:
Either chop by hand or you can use a food processor. With a food processor, mince the garlic first, then add the nuts, and then the basil, until the herbs are still rough but uniform in texture. Add the cheese and mix for about three seconds. Transfer to a bowl. If you are using the tomatoes, they get blended in by hand.

Herbs and Cottage Cheese

One of my favorite ways to eat fresh pesto is with cottage cheese on warmed and slightly crispy pita bread. This recipe makes enough for two:

Ingredients:

¼ bunch parsley
2 sprigs basil
⅛ bunch cilantro
2 cloves garlic
Salt and Pepper to Taste
2 shakes Cayenne Pepper
1 cup organic small or medium curd cottage cheese
1-2 tbsp organic cream cheese

Directions:

In a food processor, mince the garlic, and then add the parsley, basil, and cilantro or any other herbs you choose, and chop thoroughly. Add the salt and pepper and mix for two to three seconds more. Transfer the herbs to a mixing bowl. Add the cottage cheese and sour cream or cream cheese and blend well. Then add a couple of shakes of Cayenne and serve over the pita.

Pesto Pate over Fresh Bread

Ingredients:

2 cups of any combination of fresh herbs
1 clove garlic
1 cup walnuts or pecans
2–4 tablespoons extra virgin olive oil
Salt and Pepper to taste
1/2 cup finely grated Parmesan cheese

Directions:

In a food processor, start with the garlic. After it is minced, add the nuts, and then the herbs, salt, pepper, and oil. Mix into a paste. Then add the Parmesan cheese and mix for three to five seconds. Transfer to a pretty serving dish and add a sprig of parsley as a garnish. Spread over fresh rye or Italian bread.

Notes

Chapter 1: Asperger Syndrome: What It Is and What It Isn't

1. M. Kyrkou, October 2005. Health Issues and Quality of Life in Women with Intellectual Disability. *Journal of Intellectual Disability Research*, 49(Pt 10): 770–772.

2. A. J. Wakefield, S.A. Murch, A. Anthony, D.M. Casson, M. Malik, M. Berelowitz, A.P. Dhillon, M.A. Thomson, P. Harvey, A. Valentine, S.E. Davies, and J.A. Walker-Smith, February 28, 1998. Ileal-Lymphoid-Nodular Hyperplasia, Non-Specific Colitis, and Pervasive Developmental Disorder in Children. *Lancet*, 351(9103): 637–641.

3. K. Horvath, October 2002. Autistic Disorder and Gastrointestinal Disease. *Current Opinion in Pediatrics*, 14(5): 583–587.

4. H. M. Parrochio, October 2005. Differences between the Gut Microflora of Children with Autistic Spectrum Disorders and that of Healthy Children. *Journal of Medical Microbiology*, 54(Pt 10): 987–991.

5. Doris Rapp, 1991. *Is This Your Child?* (New York: W Morrow).

6. Doris Rapp, 1996. *Is This Your Child's World?* (New York: Bantam Books).

7. S. Ehlers and C. Gillberg, 1993. The Epidemiology of Asperger Syndrome: A Total Population Study. *Journal of Child Psychology and Psychiatry*, 34(8): 1327–1350.

8. L. Wing and J. Gould, 1979. Severe Impairments of Social Interaction and Associated Abnormalities in Children: Epidemiology and Classification. *Journal of Autism and Developmental Disorders*, 9: 11–29.

9. Christopher Gillberg, 2005. *Looking Up: Monthly International Autism Newsletter* (Interview), 3(12), http://www.lookingupautism.org/Articles/ChristopherGillberg.html, May 17, 2007.

10. S. Baron-Cohen, June 2006. fMRI of Parents of Children with Asperger Syndrome: A Pilot Study. *Brain and Cognition*, 61(1): 122–130.

11. E. Jansson-Verkasalo, August 2005. Similarities in the Phenotype of the Auditory Neural Substrate in Children with Asperger Syndrome and Their Parents. *European Journal of Neuroscience*, 22(4): 986–990.

12. E. Gilberg, August 2005. Asperger Syndrome: Familial and Pre- and Perinatal Factors. *Journal of Autism and Developmental Disorders*, 35(2): 159–166.

13. S. Aldred, February 2003. Plasma Amino Acid Levels in Children with Autism and Their Families. *Journal of Autism and Developmental Disorders*, 33(1): 93–97.

14. Michael Fitzgerald, 2001. Diagnosis and Differential Diagnosis of Asperger Syndrome. *Advances in Psychiatric Treatment*, 7: 310–318.

15. Doris Rapp, 1996. *Is This Your Child's World?* (New York: Bantam Books).

16. S. B. Edelson, July–August, 1998. Autism: Xenobiotic Influences. *Toxicology and Industrial Health*, 14(4): 553–563.

17. J. Bertrand, A. Mars, C. Boyle, F. Bove, M. Yearqin-Allsop, and P. Decoufle, November 2001. Prevalence of Autism in a United States Population: The Brick Township, New Jersey, Investigation. *Pediatrics*, 108(5): 1155–1161.

18. U.S. Environmental Protection Agency (EPA), February 3, 1999. Response to Recommendations from the Children's Health Protection Advisory Committee Regarding Evaluation of Existing Environmental Standards. 64(22): 5277–5284.

19. U.S. Environmental Protection Agency about Pesticides, http://www.epa.gov/pesticides/about/types.htm, May 19, 2007.

Chapter 3: What Asperger Syndrome Looks Like in an Adult

1. S. Shellenbarger, November 16, 2006. For Adults with Learning Disabilities, the Hardest Part of a Job Is Keeping It. *The Wall Street Journal*. A1, A3.

2. F. Abell, December 2005. An Experimental Investigation of the Phenomenology of Delusional Beliefs in People with Asperger Syndrome, *Autism: The International Journal of Research & Practice* 9(5): 515–531.

3. David Allen. May 5, 2006. Asperger Syndrome and Offending Behavior. *Wales 2nd International Autism Conference* (Published May 8, 2006).

Chapter 4: Face Blindness and Place Blindness—Who Are You and Where Am I Going?

1. J. Barton, M. Cherkasova, R. Hefter, T. Cox, M. O'Connor, and D. Manoach, August 2004. Are Patients with Social Developmental Disorders Prosopagnosic? Perceptual Heterogeneity in the Asperger and Socio-Emotional Processing Disorders. *Brain*, 127(Pt 8): 1706–1716.

2. Ingo Kennerknecht, August 1, 2006. First Report of Prevalence of Non-Syndromic Hereditary Prosopagnosia (HPA). *American Journal of Medical Genetics Part A*, 140(15): 1617–1622.

3. H. S. Levine, June 1977. Impairment of Facial Recognition After Closed Head Injuries of Varying Severity. *Cortex*, 13(2): 119–130.

4. A. W. Young, January 29, 1992. Face Recognition Impairments. *Philosophical Transactions of the Royal Society of London. Series B. Biological Sciences*, 335(1273): 47–53, discussion 54.

5. J. J. Barton, May 2003. Disorders of Face Perception and Recognition. *Neurological Clinician*, 21(2): 521–548.

6. B. Duchaine and K. Nakayama. 2006. Developmental Prosopagnosia: A Window to Content-Specific Face Processing. *Current Opinion in Neurobiology*, 16: 166–173.

7. J. Barton, M. Cherkasova, R. Hefter, T. Cox, M. O'Connor, and D. Manoach, August 2004. Are Patients with Social Developmental Disorders Prosopagnosic? Perceptual Heterogeneity in the Asperger and Socio-Emotional Processing Disorders. *Brain*, 127(Pt 8): 1706–1716.

8. Marlene Behrmann, June 2006. Seeing It Differently: Visual Processing in Autism. *Trends in Cognitive Sciences*. 10(6): 258–264.

9. G. Schwarzer, S. Huber, M. Gruter, T. Gruter, C. Gross, M. Hipfel, and I. Kennerknecht, June 10, 2006. Gaze Behaviour in Hereditary Prosopagnosia. *Psychological Research*

10. R. Hefter, 2005. Perception of Facial Expression and Facial Identity in Subjects with Social Developmental Disorders. *Neurology*, 65, 1620–1625.

Chapter 5: Conventional Asperger Treatment: Then and Now

1. E. Przkquelinski, November–December, 1987. Effect of Repeated Administration of Antidepressant Drugs on the Serum and Brain Concentration of Testosterone and its Metabolites. *Polish Journal of Pharmacology and Pharmacy*, 39(6): 683–689.

2. Food and Drug Administration (FDA), October 15, 2004. FDA Launches a Multi-Pronged Strategy to Strengthen Safeguards for Children Treated with Antidepressant Medications. *FDA News*, News Release P04-97.

3. S. Bell and M. Shipman, January–March, 2006. Fluoxetine Treatment and Testosterone Levels. *Annals of Clinical Psychology*, 18(1): 19–22.

4. E. Przkquelinski, November-December, 1987. Effect of Repeated Administration of Antidepressant Drugs on the Serum and Brain Concentration of Testosterone and its Metabolites. *Polish Journal of Pharmacology and Pharmacy*, 39(6): 683–689.

5. J. A. Mattes, March 1983. Growth of Hyperactive Children on Maintenance Regimen of Methylphenidate. *Archives of General Psychiatry*, 40(3): 317–321.

6. J. A. Mattes, December 1988. Methylphenidate and Growth in Hyperactive Children. A Controlled Withdrawal Study. *Archives of General Psychiatry*, 45(12): 1127–1130.

7. T. E. Wilens, February 2004. Effects of Once-Daily Osmotic-Release Methylphenidate on Blood Pressure and Heart Rate in Children with Attention-Deficit/Hyperactivity Disorder: Results from a One-Year Follow-Up Study. *Journal of Clinical Psychopharmacology*, 24(1): 36–41.

8. Pediatric Advisory Committee of the Food and Drug Administration. March 22, 2006. Hilton: Washington, DC North, 620 Perry Parkway, Gaithersburg, Maryland, 20877, http://www.fda.gov/ohrms/dockets/ac/06/transcripts/2006-4210t_01_Draft%20-%20Transcript%200322fda.htm, May 19, 2007.

9. No Author. December 17, 2004. FDA Public Health Advisory. New Warning for Strattera, http://www.fda.gov/bbs/topics/NEWS/2005/NEW01237.html.html, May 19, 2007.

10. FDA Public Health Advisory, September 29, 2005. Suicidal Thinking in Children and Adolescents Being Treated with Strattera (Atomoxetine), http://www.fda.gov/CDER/DRUG/advisory/atomoxetine.htm, May 19, 2007.

11. T. A. Henderson, September 2004. Aggression, Mania, and Hypomania Induction Associated with Atomoxetine. *Pediatrics*, 114(3): 895–896.

12. C. Krachtovil, J. Newcorn, A. Eugene, D. Duesenberg, G. Emslie, H. Quintana, E. Sarkis, K. Wagner, H. Gao, D. Michelson, and J. Biederman, September 2005. Atomoxetine Alone or Combined with Fluoxetine for Treating ADHD with Comorbid Depressive or Anxiety Symptoms. *Journal of the American Academy of Child and Adolescent Psychiatry*, 44(9): 915–924.

13. Grace E. Jackson, 2005. *Rethinking Psychiatric Drugs*. (Bloomington, Indiana: Author House, 2005), 268.

14. P. W. Troost, October 2006. Atomoxetine for Attention-Deficit/Hyperactivity Disorder Symptoms in Children with Pervasive Developmental Disorders: A Pilot Study. *Journal of Child and Adolescent Psychopharmacology* 16(5): 611–619.

15. Theodore I. Benzer, Harvard Medical School, http://www.emedicine.com/EMERG/topic339.htm, May 19, 2007

16. A. Monji, August 2004. Carbamazepine May Trigger New-Onset Epileptic Seizures in an Individual with Autism Spectrum Disorders: A Case Report. *European Psychiatry*, 19(5): 322–323.

17. J. P. Horrigan, August 1999. Guanfacine and Secondary Mania in Children. *Journal of Affective Disorders*, 54(3): 309–314.

18. Grace E. Jackson, 2005. Rethinking Psychiatric Drugs. (Bloomington, Indiana: Author House, 2005), 145.

19. Ibid.

Chapter 6: Physical Symptoms Associated with Asperger Syndrome

1. Kevin Becker, April 23, 2003. Comparative Genomics of Autism, Tourette Syndrome and Autoimmune/Inflammatory Disorders. National Institute on Aging, National Institutes of Health.

2. M. G. Welch, 2005. Brain Effects of Chronic IBD in Areas Abnormal in Autism and Treatment by Single Neuropeptides Secretin and Oxytocin. *Journal of Molecular Neuroscience*, 25(3): 259–274.

3. K. Horvath, October 2002. Autistic Disorder and Gastrointestinal Disease. *Current Opinion in Pediatrics*, 14(5): 583–587.

4. A. J. Wakefield, S.H. Murch, A. Anthony, J. Linnell, D.M. Casson, M. Malik, M. Berelowitz, A.P. Dhillon, M.A. Thomson, P. Harvey, A. Valentine, S.E. Davies, and J.A. Walker-Smith, February 28, 1998. Ileal-Lymphoid-Nodular Hyperplasia, Non-Specific Colitis, and Pervasive Developmental Disorder in Children. *Lancet*, 351(9103): 637–641.

5. K. Horvath, October 2002. Autistic Disorder and Gastrointestinal Disease. *Current Opinion in Pediatrics*, 14(5): 583–587.

6. H. M. Parrochio, October 2005. Differences between the Gut Microflora of Children with Autistic Spectrum Disorders and that of Healthy Children. *Journal of Medical Microbiology*, 54(Pt 10): 987–991.

7. Kerry Bone, 2000. *Principle and Practice of Phytotherapy*. Churchill Livingstone: Sydney.

8. W. Fabry, January–February, 1996. Fungistatic and Fungicidal Activity of East African Medicinal Plants. *Mycoses*, 39(1–2): 67–70.

9. B. M. Csaba, March 2006. Anxiety as an Independent Cardiovascular Risk. *Neuropsychopharmacologica Hungarica*, 8(1): 5–11.

10. H. Uyarel, February 2006. Effects of Anxiety on QT Dispersion in Healthy Young Men. *Acta Cardiologica*, 61(1): 83–87.

11. M. Esler, July 2006. The Neuronal Noradrenaline Transporter, Anxiety and Cardiovascular Disease. *Journal of Psychopharmacology*, 20(4 Suppl): 60–66.

Chapter 7: What You Eat Affects How You Act

1. R. Molteni, R. J. Barnard, Z. Ying, C.K. Roberts, and F. Gomez-Pinella,, 2000. A High-Fat, Refined Sugar Diet Reduces Hippocampal Brain-Derived Neurotrophic Factor, Neuronal Plasticity, and Learning. *Neuroscience*, 112, 803–814.

2. A. Westover, 2002. A Cross-National Relationship between Sugar Consumption and Major Depression? *Depression and Anxiety* 16(3): 118–120.

3. C. Colantuoni, J. Schwenker, J. McCarthy, P. Rada, B. Ladeheim, J.L. Cadet, G.J. Schwartz, T.H. Moran, and B.G. Hoebel, November 16, 2001. Excessive Sugar Intake Alters Binding to Dopamine and Mu-Opioid Receptors in the Brain. *NeuroReport*, 12(16): 3549–3552.

4. P. Silviera, November 2000. Interaction between Repeated Restraint Stress and Concomitant Midazolam Administration on Sweet Food Ingestion in Rats. *Brazilian Journal of Medical and Biological Research*, 33(11): 1343–1350.

5. T. W. Jones, W.P. Borq, S.D. Boulware, G. McCarthy, R.S. Sherwin, and W.V. Tamborlane, 1995. Enhanced Adrenomedullary Response and Increased Susceptibility to Neuroglycopenia: Mechanisms Underlying the Adverse Effects of Sugar Ingestion in Healthy Children. *Journal of Pediatrics*, 126: 171–177.

6. Lars Lien et al., 2006. Consumption of Soft Drinks and Hyperactivity, Mental Distress, and Conduct Problems among Adolescents in Oslo, Norway. *American Journal of Public Health*, 96(10): 1815–1820.

7. C. Erlanson-Albertsson, May 23–29, 2005. Sugar Triggers Our Reward-System. Sweets Release Opiates Which Stimulates the Appetite for Sucrose—Insulin Can Depress It. *Lakartidningen*, 102(21): 1620–1622, 1625, 1627.

8. C. Jayasinghe July 16, 2003. Phenolics Composition and Antioxidant Activity of Sweet Basil (*Ocimum basilicum L.*), *Journal of Agriculture and Food Chemistry*, 51(15): 4442–4449.

9. S. Singh, March 1999. Evaluation of Gastric Anti-Ulcer Activity of Fixed Oil of Ocimum Basilicum Linn and Its Possible Mechanism of Action. *Indian Journal of Experimental Biology*, 37(3): 253–2537.

10. O. Ozsoy-Sacan, R. Yanardaq, H. Orak, Y. Ozgey, A. Yarat and Tunali, March 8, 2006. Effects of Parsley (Petroselinum crispum) Extract versus Glibornuride on the Liver of Streptozotocin-Induced Diabetic Rats. *Journal of Ethnopharmacology*, 104(1–2): 175–181.

11. L. Jirovetz, June 18, 2003. Composition, Quality Control, and Antimicrobial Activity of the Essential Oil of Long-Time Stored Dill (Anethum Graveolens L.) Seeds from Bulgaria. *Journal of Agriculture and Food Chemistry*, 51(13): 3854–3857.

12. H. Hosseinzadeh, December 19, 2002. Effects of Anethum Graveolens L. Seed Extracts on Experimental Gastric Irritation Models in Mice. *BMC Pharmacology*, 2: 21.

13. J. Smith, C. Terpening, S. Schmidt, and J. Gums, June 2001. Relief of Fibromyalgia Symptoms Following Discontinuation of Dietary Excitotoxins. *Annuals of Pharmacotherapy*, 35(6): 702–706.

14. Y.F. Sasaki, S. Kawaquchi, A. Kamaya, M. Ohshita, K. Kabasawa, K. Iwama, K. Taniquchi, and S. Tsuda, August 26, 2002. The Comet Assay with 8 Mouse Organs: Results with 39 Currently Used Food Additives. *Mutation Research*, 519(1–2): 103–119.

15. S.W. Mann, M.M. Yuschak, S.J. Aymes, P. Aughton, and J.P. Finn, 2000. A Combined Chronic Toxicity/Carcinogenicity Study of Sucralose in Sprague-Dawley Rats. *Food Chemical Toxicology*, 38(Suppl. 2): S71–S89.

16. I.M. Baird, N.W. Shephard, R.J. Merritt, and G. Hildick-Smith, 2000. Repeated Dose Study of Sucralose Tolerance in Human Subjects. *Food Chemical Toxicology*. 38(Suppl. 2): S123–S129.

17. Joseph Mercola, 2006. *Sweet Deception* (Nashville, TN: Thomas Nelson Inc.).

18. F. X. Qin, August 2002. Impaired Inactivation of Digestive Proteases by Deconjugated Bilirubin: The Possible Mechanism for Inflammatory Bowel Disease. *Medical Hypotheses*, 59(2): 159–163.

19. G. Torres de Mercau, N. Riviera de Martinez Villa, H. Vitalone, G. Mercau, S. Gamundi, N. Martinez Riera, and N. Soria, 1997. Sodium Saccharin Effect on the Mice Large Intestine. *Acta Gastroenterol Latinoam*, 27(2): 63–65.

20. G. Torres de Mercau, N. Riviera de Martinez Villa, G. Mercau, N. Martinez Riera, N. Soria de Santos, and H. Vitalone, 1995. Changes in Cytomembrane and Surface Cells of the Large Intestine Resulting from the Action of Sweetening Agents. *Acta Gastroenterol Latinoam*, 25(1): 35–39.

21. E. M. Garland, October 1993. Effects of Dietary Iron and Folate Supplementation on the Physiological Changes Produced in Weaning Rats by Sodium Saccharin Exposure. *Food and Chemical Toxicology*, 31(10): 689–699.

22. L. A. Ferri, W. Alvez-Do-Prado, S.S. Yamada, S. Gazola, M.R. Batista, and R.B. Bazotte, September 2006. Investigation of the Antihypertensive Effect of Oral Crude Stevioside in Patients with Mild Essential Hypertension. *Phytotherapy Research*, 20(9): 732–736.

23. M. H. Hsieh, P. Chan, Y.M. Sue, J.C. Liu, T.H. Liang, T.Y. Luang, B. Tomlinson, M.S. Chow, P.F. Kao, and Y.J. Chen, November 2003. Efficacy and Tolerability of Oral Stevioside in Patients with Mild Essential Hypertension: A Two-Year, Randomized, Placebo-Controlled Study. *Clinical Therapy*, 25(11): 2797–2808.

24. P. A. Chan, September 2000. Double-Blind Placebo-Controlled Study of the Effectiveness and Tolerability of Oral Stevioside in Human Hypertension. *British Journal of Clinical Pharmacology*, 50(3): 215–220.

25. H. Mineo, June 2002. Sugar Alcohols Enhance Calcium Transport from Rat Small and Large Intestine Epithelium In Vitro. *Digestive Diseases and Sciences*, 47(6): 1326–1333.

26. Ing Zbynek Polesny, 2002 *Tropical and Subtropical Plants with Sweetening Properties*. Czech University of Agriculture: Prague.

27. Fang Fang Song, 2006. A Natural Sweetener, *Momordica grosvenori*, Attenuates the Imbalance of Cellular Immune Functions in Alloxan-Induced Diabetic Mice. *Phytotherapy Research*, 20(7): 552–560.

28. S. Bashir, K. H. Janbaz, Q. Jabeen, and A. H. Gilani, October 2006. Studies on Spasmogenic and Spasmolytic Activities of Calendula Officinalis Flowers. *Phytotherapy Research*, 20(10): 906–910.

29. E. Jimenez-Medina, A. Garcia-Lora, L. Paco, I. Algarra, A. Collado, and F. Garrido, May 5, 2006. A New Extract of the Plant Calendula Officinalis Produces a Dual In Vitro Effect: Cytotoxic Anti-Tumor Activity and Lymphocyte Activation. *BioMed Central Cancer*, 6: 119.

30. V. Duran, M. Matik, M. Jovanovc, N. Mimica, Z. Gaginov, M. Poljacki, and P. Boza, 2005. Results of the Clinical Examination of an Ointment with Marigold (Calendula Officinalis) Extract in the Treatment of Venous Leg Ulcers. *International Journal of Tissue Reactions*, 27(3): 101–106.

31. A. Iauk, A.M. Lo Bue, I. Milazzo, A. Rapizarda, and G. Blandino, June 2003. Antibacterial Activity of Medicinal Plant Extracts against Periodontopathic Bacteria. *Phytotherapy Research*, 17(6): 599–604.

32. A. Cardosova, July 2006. Antioxidant Activity of Medicinal Plant Polysaccharides. *Fitoterapia*, 77(5): 367–373.

33. A. Herald, July–December, 2003. Antioxidant Properties of Some Hydroalcoholic Plant Extracts with Anti-Inflammatory Activity. *Roumanian Archives of Microbiology and Immunology*, 62(3–4): 217–227.

34. M. T. Khayyal, 2001. Antiulcerogenic Effect of Some Gastrointestinally Acting Plant Extracts and Their Combination. *Arzneimittelforshung*, 51(7): 545–553.

35. I. Dadalioqlu, December 29, 2004. Chemical Compositions and Antibacterial Effects of Essential Oils of Turkish Oregano (Origanum Minutiflorum), Bay Laurel (Laurus nobilis), Spanish Lavender (Lavandula Stoechas L.), and Fennel (Foeniculum Vulgare) on Common Foodborne Pathogens. *Journal of Agriculture and Food Chemistry*, 52(26): 8255–8260.

36. I. Chakurski, 1981. Treatment of Chronic Colitis with an Herbal Combination. *Vutr. Boles*, 20(6): 51–54.

37. Puneet Gupta, 2000. Is Lactobacillus GG Helpful in Children with Crohn's Disease? Results of a Preliminary, Open-Label Study. *Journal of Pediatric Gastroenterology & Nutrition*, 31(4): 453–457.

Chapter 8: How the Environment Affects Asperger Syndrome

1. U.S. FDA, 1990. Neurotoxicity: Identifying and Controlling Poisons of the Nervous System. U.S. Congress, Office of Technology Assessment (OTA-BA-436). Washington, DC: U.S. Government Printing Office.

2. Doris Rapp, 1996. *Is This Your Child's World?* (New York: Bantam Books).

3. K. Horvath and J.A. Perman, October 2002. Autistic Disorder and Gastrointestinal Disease. *Current Opinion in Pediatrics*, 14(5): 583–587.

4. B. I. Cohen, December 2002. The Significance of Ammonia/Gamma-Aminobutyric Acid (GABA) Ratio for Normality and Liver Disorders. *Medical Hypotheses*, 59(6): 757–758.

5. A. Wakefield, April 2002. Review Article: The Concept of Entero-Colonic Encephalopathy, Autism and Opioid Receptor Ligands. *Alimentary Pharmacology and Therapeutics*, 16(4): 663–674.

6. Abram Ber, 1983. Neutralization of Phenolic (Aromatic) Food Compounds in a Holistic General Practice. *The Journal of Orthomolecular Psychiatry*, 12(4): 283–291.

7. J.H. Kim, B.C. Campbell, J. Yu, N. Mahoney, K.L. Chan, R.J. Molyneux, D. Bhatnaqar, and T.E. Cleveland, June 2005. Examination of Fungal Stress Response Genes Using Saccharomyces Cerevisiae as a Model System. USDA (U.S. Department of Agriculture). *Applied Microbiology and Biotechnology*, 67(6): 807–815.

8. L. Morello, August 1, 2006. EPA to End Use of Lindane. Environment and Energy News, http://www.headlice.org/lindane/new/080106_end_use_lindane.html and http://www.headlice.org/lindane/index.htm, May19, 2007.

9. U.S. EPA. about Pesticides, http://www.epa.gov/pesticides/about/types.htm.

10. U.S. Congress Office of Technology Assessment. 1990. Neurotoxicity: Identifying and Controlling Poisons of the Nervous System, OTA-BA-436. Washington, DC: U.S. Government Printing Office.

11. E. D. Caldes, 2006. Probabilistic Assessment of the Cumulative Acute Exposure to Organophosphorus and Carbamate Insecticides in the Brazilian Diet. *Toxicology*, 222(2006) 132–142.

12. Office of Technology Assessment, April 1990. Neurotoxicity: Identifying and Controlling Poisons of the Nervous System, *United States Congress*.

13. M. O'Brian, 1990. Are Pesticides Taking Away the Ability of Our Children to Learn? http://eap.mcgill.ca/MagRack/JPR/jpr_head.htm.

14. W. P. Porter, January–March, 1999. Endocrine, Immune, and Behavioral Effects of Aldicarb (Carbamate), Atrazine (Triazine) and Nitrate (Fertilizer) Mixtures at Groundwater Concentrations. *Toxicology and Industrial Health*, 15(1–2): 133–150.

15. M. Carbonaro, September 11, 2002. Modulation of Antioxidant Compounds in Organic versus Conventional Fruit (Peach, Prunus Persica L., and Pear, Pyrus Communis L.). *Journal of Agricultural and Food Chemistry*, 50(19): 5458–5462.

16. G. Lombardii-Boccia, January 14, 2004. Nutrients and Antioxidant Molecules in Yellow Plums (Prunus Domestica L.) from Conventional and Organic Productions: A Comparative Study. *Journal of Agricultural and Food Chemistry*, 52(1): 90–94.

17. M. E. Olsson, February 22, 2006. Antioxidant Levels and Inhibition of Cancer Cell Proliferation In Vitro by Extracts from Organically and Conventionally Cultivated Strawberries. *Journal of Agricultural and Food Chemistry*, 54(4): 1248–1255.

18. C. Caris-Veyrat, October 20, 2004. Influence of Organic versus Conventional Agricultural Practice on the Antioxidant Microconstituent Content of Tomatoes and Derived Purees; Consequences on Antioxidant Plasma Status in Humans. *Journal of Agricultural and Food Chemistry*, 52(21): 6503–6509.

19. D. K. Asami, February 26, 2003. Comparison of the Total Phenolic and Ascorbic Acid Content of Freeze-Dried and Air-Dried Marionberry, Strawberry, and Corn Grown Using Conventional, Organic, and Sustainable Agricultural Practices. *Journal of Agricultural and Food Chemistry*, 51(5): 1237–1241.

20. V. Worthington, April 2001. Nutritional Quality of Organic versus Conventional Fruits, Vegetables, and Grains. *Journal of Alternative and Complementary Medicine*, 7(2): 161–173.

21. Y. F. Sasaki, August 26, 2002. The Comet Assay with 8 Mouse Organs: Results with 39 Currently Used Food Additives. *Mutation Research*, 519(1–2): 103–119.

22. R. Schoental, February 1985. Fusarial Mycotoxins and Behaviour: Possible Implications for Psychiatric Disorder. *The British Journal of Psychiatry*, 146: 115–119.

23. W. J. Walsh, A. Usman, and J. Tarpey, May 2001. Disordered Metal Metabolism in a Large Autism Population, Proceedings of the American Psychiatric Association. *New Research: Abstract*, NR109, New Orleans, Louisiana.

24. Institute for Vaccine Safety, 2006. Thimerosal Content in Some U.S. Licensed Vaccines. *John Hopkins Bloomberg School of Public Health*, http://www.vaccinesafety.edu/thi-table.htm.

25. National Center for Environmental Health Division of Laboratory Sciences Atlanta, Georgia 30341-3724, July 2005. Third National Report on Human Exposure to Environmental Chemicals Department of Health and Human Services. Centers for Disease Control and Prevention, http://www.cdc.gov/exposurereport/3rd/pdf/thirdreport.pdf. NCEH Pub. No. 05-0570.

26. David Kirby, 2005. *Evidence of Harm. Mercury in Vaccines and the Autism Epidemic: A Medical Controversy.* New York: St. Martin's Press.

27. P. Carta, August 2003. Sub-Clinical Neurobehavioral Abnormalities Associated with Low Level of Mercury Exposure through Fish Consumption. *Neurotoxicology*, 24(4–5): 617–623.

28. C. Sanfeliu, 2003. Neurotoxicity of Organomercurial Compounds. *Neurotoxicology Research*, 5(4): 283–305.

29. L. Raymond and N. Ralston, November 2004. Mercury: Selenium Interactions and Health Implications. *SMDJ Seychelles Medical and Dental Journal*, Special Issue, 7(1): 72–77.

30. See http://www.epa.gov/safewater/lead/, U.S. Environmental Protection Agency.

31. Autism Research Institute, 2005. Treatment Options for Mercury/Metal Toxicity in Autism and Related Developmental Disabilities: Consensus Position Paper, http://www.autismwebsite.com/ari/dan/heavymetals.pdf.

32. Hall and Winkvist. A Treatment for the Removal of Metal and Environmental Toxins, http://www.positivehealth.com/permit/Articles/Dentist/hall11.htm.

33. E. O. Uthos, February 2005. Dietary Arsenic Affects Dimethylhydrazine-Induced Aberrant Crypt Formation and Hepatic Global DNA Methylation and DNA Methyltransferase Activity in Rats. *Biological Trace Element Research*, 103(2): 133–145.

34. S. Samuel, January 15, 2005. Protein Oxidative Damage in Arsenic Induced Rat Brain: Influence of DL-Alpha-Lipoic Acid. *Toxicology Letters*, 155(1): 27–34.

35. K. K. Das, 2006. Effect of L-Ascorbic Acid on Nickel-Induced Alterations in Serum Lipid Profiles and Liver Histopathology in Rats. *Journal of Basic Physiology and Pharmacology*, 17(1): 29–44.

36. M. Modi, 2006. Co-Administration of Zinc And N-Acetylcysteine Prevents Arsenic-Induced Tissue Oxidative Stress in Male Rats. *Journal of Trace Elements in Medicine and Biology*, 20(3): 197–204.

37. Kerry Bone, 2001. The Effect of Herbs on Liver Detoxification. *The British Journal of Phytotherapy*, 5(4) 176–183.

38. K. L. Wilde, August 2006. The Effect of pH on the Uptake and Toxicity of Copper and Zinc in a Tropical Freshwater Alga (Chlorella sp.). *Archives of Environmental Contamination and Toxicology*, 51(2): 174–185.

39. S. S. Ahluwalia, September 2007. Microbial and Plant Derived Biomass for Removal of Heavy Metals from Wastewater. *Bioresource Technology*, 98(12): 2243-57.

40. N. Mallick, May 2004. Copper-Induced Oxidative Stress in the Chlorophycean Microalga Chlorella Vulgaris: Response of the Antioxidant System. *Journal of Plant Physiology*, 161(5): 591–597.

41. S. Bolkent, December 2004. Effects of Parsley (Petroselinum Crispum) on the Liver of Diabetic Rats: A Morphological and Biochemical Study. *Phytotherapy Research*, 18(12): 996–999.

42. S. Daniel, February 2004. Through Metal Binding, Curcumin Protects against Lead- and Cadmium-Induced Lipid Peroxidation in Rat Brain Homogenates and against Lead-Induced Tissue Damage in Rat Brain. *Journal of Inorganic Biochemistry*, 98(2): 266–275.

43. F. Haunchman, 2003. Drinking Water Research Program: Multi-Year Plan. Office of Research and Development U.S. Environmental Protection Agency, http://www.epa.gov/osp/myp/dw.pdf.

44. A. Veraldi, December 2006. Immunotoxic Effects of Chemicals: A Matrix for Occupational and Environmental Epidemiological Studies. *American Journal of Industrial Medicine*, 49(12): 1046–1055.

45. B.A. Sorq, March 2001. Repeated Formaldehyde Effects in an Animal Model for Multiple Chemical Sensitivity. *Annals of the New York Academy of Sciences*, 933: 57–67.

46. M. Geise, 1994. Detoxification of Formaldehyde by the Spider Plant (Chlorophytum comosum L.) and by Soybean (Glycine Max L.) Cell-Suspension Cultures. *Plant Physiology*, 104(4): 1301–1309.

47. T. Oyabu, 2003. Purification Characteristics of Golden Pothos for Atmospheric Gasoline. *International Journal of Phytoremediation*, 5(3): 267–276.

48. F. Hollowich, July 1977. The Effect of Natural and Artificial Light via the Eye on the Hormonal and Metabolic Balance of Man. *Klin Monatsbl Augenheilkunde*, 171(1): 98–104.

49. R.S. Coleman, F. Frankel, E. Ritvo, and B.J. Freeman, June 1976. The Effects of Fluorescent and Incandescent Illumination upon Repetitive Behaviors in Autistic Children. *Journal of Autism and Childhood Schizophrenia*, 6(2): 157–162.

50. E. Gluskin, 2006. The Autistic Vision Problem with Light from Fluorescent Lamps Explained in Terms of Coherence and Phase Shift. *Medical Hypotheses*, 66(1): 207–208.

51. R. Becker, *Cross Current: the Promise of Electromedicine, the Perils of Electropollution.* (New York: Penguin Group. 1990).

52. J. Ott, 1985–1991. Series of Seven Articles in Seven Issues. *International Journal for Biosocial Research.*

Chapter 9: Deer in the Headlights—Dealing with Anxiety, Depression, and Sleep

1. S. Baron-Cohen, June 2006. fMRI of Parents of Children with Asperger Syndrome: A Pilot Study. *Brain and Cognition*, 61(1): 122–130.

2. A. Gomez-Caminero, September–October, 2005. Does Panic Disorder Increase the Risk of Coronary Heart Disease? A Cohort Study of a National Managed Care Database. *Psychosomatic Medicine*, 67(5): 688–691.

3. B. Gustafsson, K. Tommeras, I. Nordrum, J. Loennechen, A. Bursvik, E. Solligard, R. Fossmark, I. Bakke, U. Syversen, and H. Waldum. 2005. Long-Term Serotonin Administration Induces Heart Valve Disease in Rats. *Circulation*, 111: 1517–1522.

4. N. Gulta, 2006. Effect of Yoga-Based Lifestyle Intervention on State and Trait Anxiety. *Indian Journal of Physiology and Pharmacology*, 50(1): 41–47.

5. Joan Mathews Larson, 1999. *Depression-Free, Naturally.* (New York: Ballantine Publishing Group).

6. R. J. Boerner, H. Sommer, W. Berger, U. Kahn, U. Schmidt, and M. Mannel, 2003. Kava-Kava Extract LI 150 is as Effective as Opipramol and Buspirone in Generalised Anxiety Disorder—An 8-Week Randomized, Double-Blind Multi-Centre Clinical Trial in 129 Out-Patients. *Phytomedicine: International Journal of Phytotherapy and Phytopharmacology*, 10(Suppl 4): 38–49.

7. F. P. Geier and T. Konstantinowicz, 2004. Kava Treatment in Patients with Anxiety. *Phytotherapy Research*, 18: 297–300.

8. D. O. Kennedy, W. Little, and A. B. Scholey, 2004. Attenuation of Laboratory-Induced Stress in Humans After Acute Administration of *Melissa Officinalis* (Lemon Balm). *Psychosomatic Medicine*, 66: 607–613.

9. D. O. Kennedy, G. Wake, S. Savelev, N.T. Tildesley, E.K. Perry, K.A. Wesnes, and A.B. Scholey, October 2003. Modulation of Mood and Cognitive Performance Following Acute Administration of Single Doses of *Melissa Officinalis* (Lemon Balm) with Human CNS Nicotinic and Muscarinic Receptor-Binding Properties. *Neuropsychopharmacology,* 28(10): 1871–1881.

10. D. O. Kennedy, W. Little, C.F. Haskell, and A.B. Scholey, February 2006. Anxiolytic Effects of a Combination of Melissa Officinalis and Valeriana Officinalis during Laboratory Induced Stress. *Phytotherapy Research,* 20(2): 96–102.

11. S. Akhondzadel, H.R. Naghavi, M. Vazirian, A. Sahayeganpour, H. Rashidi, and M. Khani, October 2003. Passionflower in the Treatment of Generalized Anxiety. *Journal of Clinical Pharmacy and Therapeutics,* 26(5): 363–367.

Chapter 10: Homeopathy: A Giant Leap Forward

1. K. Linde, N. Clausius, G. Ramirez, D. Melchart, F. Eitel, L.V. Hedges, and W.B. Jonas, September 1997. Are the Clinical Effects of Homeopathy Placebo Effects? A Meta-Analysis of Palcebo-controlled Trials. *Lancet,* 350(9081): 834–843.

2. J. Kleijnen, P. Knipschild, and G. ter Riert, April 1991. Clinical Trials of Homeopathy. *British Medical Journal,* 302(6780): 316–323.

3. J. Jacobs, L.M. Jimenez, S.S. Gloyd, J.L. Gale, and D. Crothers, May 1994. Treatment of Acute Childhood Diarrhea with Homeopathic Medicine: A Randomized Clinical Trial in Nicaragua. *Pediatrics,* 93(5): 719–725.

Chapter 11: What You Can Do Right Now

1. N. Gupta, 2006. Effect of Yoga-Based Lifestyle Intervention on State and Trait Anxiety. *Indian Journal of Physiology and Pharmacology,* 50(1): 41–47.

2. A. Michalson, December 2005. Rapid Stress Reduction and Anxiolysis among Distressed Women as a Consequence of a Three-Month Intensive Yoga Program. *Medical Science Monitor,* 11(12): CR555–CR561.

3. G. Kirkwood, December 2005. Yoga for Anxiety: A Systematic Review of the Research Evidence. *British Journal of Sports Medicine,* 39(12): 884–891.

4. A. Woolery, March–April, 2004. A Yoga Intervention for Young Adults with Elevated Symptoms of Depression. *Alternative Therapies Health Journal,* 10(2): 60–63.

5. T. Takahashi, T. Murata, T. Hamada, M. Omori, H. Kosaka, M. Kikuchi, H. Yoshida, and Y. Wada, February 2005. Changes in EEG and Autonomic Nervous Activity during Meditation and their Association with Personality Traits. *The International Journal of Psychophysiology,* 55(2): 199–207.

6. J. C. Tsao, 2003. Fear of Loss of Vigilance: Development and Preliminary Validation of a Self-Report Instrument. *Depression and Anxiety,* 18(4): 177–186.

Selected Bibliography

Appleton, Nancy, *Lick the Sugar Habit*. Garden City Park, NY: Avery Publishing Group, 1996.

Becker, Robert O., *Cross Current*. New York: Penguin Group, 1990.

Blaylock, Russell, *Excitotoxins: The Taste that Kills*. Sante Fe, New Mexico: Health Press, 1997.

Braverman, E.R., *The Healing Nutrients Within*. New Canaan, CT: Keats Publishing, 1997.

———. *The Edge Effect*. New York: Sterling Publishing Co., 2004.

Colborn, Theo, *Our Stolen Future*. New York: Penguin Books, 1997.

Exkorn, Karen Siff, *The Autism Source Book*. New York: HarperCollins Publishers, 2005.

Hersey, Jane, *Why Can't My Child Behave? The Feingold Diet Updated for Today's Busy Families*. Alexandria, VA: Pear Tree Press, 1999.

Jackson, Grace E., *Rethinking Psychiatric Drugs—A Guide for Informed Consent*. Bloomington, IN: AuthorHouse, 2005.

Kirby, David, *Evidence of Harm. Mercury in Vaccines and the Autism Epidemic: A Medical Controversy*. New York: St. Martin's Press, 2005.

Kranowitz, Carol Stock, *The Out-of-Sync Child*. New York: The Berkeley Publishing Group, 2005.

Larson, Joan Mathews, *Depression-Free, Naturally*. New York: Ballantine Publishing Group, 1999.

Lesser, Michael, *The Brain Chemistry Diet*. New York: G.P. Putnam's Sons, 2002.

Rapp, Doris J., *Is This Your Child's World?* New York: Bantam Books, 1996.

Simontacchi, Carol, *The Crazy Makers: How the Food Industry Is Destroying our Brains and Harming Our Children*. New York: Jeremy P. Tarcher/Putnam, 2000.

Wolverton, B.C., *How to Grow Fresh Air: 50 Houseplants that Purify Your Home or Office*. New York: Penguin Books, 1996.

Index

About the Author and Series Editor

SUZANNE C. LAWTON, N.D., is a family practitioner in Oregon where she uses diet, nutritional supplements, homeopathy, herbs, and sometimes conventional medicine to treat disease. Her specialty is neurological conditions including Asperger Syndrome, ADHD, and other learning disorders.

CHRIS D. MELETIS, N.D., is Senior Series Editor. He is the Executive Director for the Institute for Healthy Aging, www.TheIHA.org, a non-profit organization dedicated to educating the public, media, and professional community on scientific approaches to enhancing healthy aging. He was chosen for the Naturopathic Physician of the Year Award for 2003–2004 by the American Association of Naturopathic Physicians. He is an international lecturer, a radio personality, and an educator of medical doctors, nurses, pharmacists, and the allied healthcare fields. He has authored ten books on natural health topics.